O P M L

OXFORD PAIN MANAGEMENT LIBRARY

Neuropathic Pain

Editor

Dr Michael I. Bennett

Senior Clinical Lecturer and Consultant in
Palliative Medicine,
University of Leeds and St. Gemma's Hospice,
Leeds, UK.

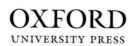

OXFORD
UNIVERSITY PRESS

OXFORD
UNIVERSITY PRESS

Great Clarendon Street, Oxford OX2 6DP

Oxford University Press is a department of the University of Oxford.
It furthers the University's objective of excellence in research, scholarship,
and education by publishing worldwide in

Oxford New York

Auckland Cape Town Dar es Salaam Hong Kong Karachi
Kuala Lumpur Madrid Melbourne Mexico City Nairobi
New Delhi Shanghai Taipei Toronto

With offices in

Argentina Austria Brazil Chile Czech Republic France Greece
Guatemala Hungary Italy Japan Poland Portugal Singapore
South Korea Switzerland Thailand Turkey Ukraine Vietnam

Oxford is a registered trade mark of Oxford University Press
in the UK and in certain other countries

Published in the United States
by Oxford University Press Inc., New York

© Oxford University Press, 2006

British Library Cataloguing in Publication Data

Data available

Library of Congress Cataloging in Publication Data

Data available

Typeset by Newgen Imaging Systems (P) Ltd, Chennai, India
Printed in the United Kingdom
on acid-free paper by CPI Bath Press

ISBN 0–19–921569–3   978–0–19–921569–0

10 9 8 7 6 5 4 3 2 1

Contents

Part 2 – **Treatment**

Contributors

Vivienne Barros D'Sa
Specialist Registar in Palliative
Medicine
Leeds Teaching Hospitals Trust,
Seacroft Hospital
York Road
Leeds
LS14 6UH

Michael I. Bennett
Senior Clinical Lecturer,
University of Leeds
Consultant in Palliative Medicine
St Gemma's Hospice
329, Harrogate Road
Leeds
LS17 6QD

David Bowsher
Emeritus Hon. Consultant Neu-
rologist (Pain Relief)
Former Reader in Neurological
Sciences, University of Liverpool
Pain Relief Foundation
Clinical Sciences Centre
University Hospital Aintree
Lower Lane
Liverpool
L9 7AL

Dudley Bush
Consultant Anaesthetist and
Clinical Director
Pain Management Service
L ward
Seacroft Hospital
York Road
Leeds
LS14 6UH

S. José Closs
Professor of Nursing Research
School of Healthcare
Baines Wing
University of Leeds
Leeds
LS2 9UT

Marie T. Fallon
Reader in Palliative Medicine
University of Edinburgh
Edinburgh Cancer Centre
Western General Hospital
Crewe Road
Edinburgh
EH4 2XU

Cameron Fergus
Specialist Registrar in Palliative
Medicine
Edinburgh Cancer Centre
Western General Hospital
Crewe Road
Edinburgh
EH4 2XU

Irene J. Higginson
Professor of Palliative Care and
Policy
Department of Palliative Care
and Policy, Weston Education
Centre, Kings College London

Mark Johnson
Professor of Pain and Analgesia
Faculty of Health
Leeds Metropolitan University
Calverley Street, Leeds
LS1 3HE

Gary McCleane
Consultant in Pain Management
Rampark Pain Centre
2 Rampark
Dromore Road
Lurgan N. Ireland
BT66 7JH

Henry J. McQuay
Professor of Pain Relief
University of Oxford
Pain Relief Unit
Churchill Hospital Oxford
OX3 7LJ

Fliss E. Murtagh
Research Training Fellow
Department of Palliative Care
and Policy
Weston Education Centre
Kings College London

Tim Nash
Honorary Senior Lecturer
Department of Neuroscience,
University of Liverpool
Consultant in Pain Medicine
Walton Centre for Neurology
and Neurosurgery
Lower Lane Fazakerley
Liverpool,
L9 7LJ

Brian A. Simpson
Consultant Neurosurgeon
Department of Neurosurgery
University Hospital of Wales
Heath Park, Cardiff
CF14 4XW

Karen H. Simpson
Consultant in Pain
Management and Senior

Clinical Lecturer
Leeds Teaching Hospitals
Trust, Seacroft Hospital
York Road
Leeds
LS14 6UH

Blair H. Smith
Reader in General Practice
Department of General
Practice and Primary Care
University of Aberdeen
Foresterhill Health Centre
Westburn Road
Aberdeen AB25 2AY

Nicola Torrance
Research Fellow
Department of General
Practice and Primary Care
University of Aberdeen
Foresterhill Health Centre
Westburn Road
Aberdeen AB25 2AY

Catherine E. Urch
Honorary Senior Lecturer
UCL and Imperial College
Consultant in Palliative
Medicine
St Mary's and Royal Brompton
Hospitals
Department of Palliative Care
St Mary's Hospital
Praed Street Paddington
W2 1NY

Phillip Wiffen
Co-ordinating Editor
Cochrane Pain & Palliative
Care Group, Pain Relief Unit
Churchill Hospital, Oxford
OX3 7LJ

Preface

Chronic pain is a huge public health issue. In the UK alone, around a third of adults have some type of chronic pain and estimates suggest that as many as one in five of these adults will have symptoms of neuropathic pain. Compared with other types of pain, neuropathic pain is frequently thought of as harder to treat, often results in poorer quality of life, and is an under-recognized chronic disabling condition.

The Oxford Pain Management Library book *Neuropathic Pain* aims to be a concise companion for health care professionals across the range of primary care, and medical and surgical specialties. It is to these professionals that patients with neuropathic pain present, often repeatedly, before accurate diagnosis is made and appropriate management is started. The problem in practice is that most patients are not textbook lists of symptoms and signs, and the presentation of chronic pain in particular takes some analysis. On top of this is the sobering fact that with current treatments, only 30–50% of patients with neuropathic pain experience meaningful improvement in pain.

I hope that this book goes some way to improving recognition of neuropathic pain and reducing delays for patients in obtaining effective treatment. Alongside chapters on traditional areas relevant to neuropathic pain management, there are chapters covering emerging areas such as the epidemiology of neuropathic pain, the role of verbal description in pain assessment, and, not least, a chapter on the experiences of patients living with neuropathic pain drawn from focus group research. Each chapter summarizes up-to-date research literature in a style that has direct clinical application.

I am indebted to all the contributors to this book for their support and willingness to share their expertise. Inevitably, there will be some aspects of neuropathic pain and its management that readers may feel have been left out or overemphasized. That is entirely down to me. However, I believe that the approach taken will enable readers to gain greater insights and feel more confident when dealing with patients with neuropathic pain.

Michael Bennett
January 2006

Part 1

The patient

Chapter 1

Theories, history, and current taxonomy

Michael I. Bennett

> **Key points**
>
> - Pain is a complex experience of somatic mechanisms and psychological influences (affective and cognitive) and, as such, is always subjective in nature.
> - The nervous system is capable of substantial plasticity; it can change structure and function in response to development, injury, or experience.
> - Nociceptive pain is normal activation of pain pathways.
> - Neuropathic pain is pain that is initiated or caused by a primary lesion or dysfunction of the nervous system (abnormal activation of pain pathways).
> - Pain is usually classified by mechanism (nociceptive or neuropathic), context (physiological or pathological), and location (somatic, visceral, etc.).

1.1 Theories of pain

1.1.1 Pre-renaissance

Theories of pain date to ancient civilizations where pain was thought to be inflicted by gods or due to imbalances in 'vital energies' or 'body humours'. At this time, Aristotle proposed that the heart was the centre of sensation, and thus pain was an affective quality. Hippocrates, however, viewed the brain as the centre of sensation. Some 2000 years later, Descartes in the early seventeenth century described nerves as tubes containing threads, each connecting an area of skin directly to the brain, the seat of sensation. These threads transmitted signals in a 'hard-wired' fashion.

1.1.2 Early science

By the late nineteenth century, two distinct pain theories had emerged. The first proposed that pain is a specific sensation served by dedicated nerves independent of other sensations. This subsequently became known as the 'specificity theory'. A second pain theory, the 'summation theory', was proposed shortly after which suggested that pain was the product of any sensory modality given a stimulus of sufficient intensity. The earlier view of pain as an affective quality remained until a new theory of pain emerged in the 1950s. This 'sensory interaction theory' incorporated two components: the sensation of pain (dependent on physiological processes) and the reaction to it (dependent on cognitive and affective processes). This theory proposed the involvement of two systems in pain transmission. One consisted of slowly conducting small fibres whose activation produced painful sensations. The other consisted of faster-conducting larger fibres whose activation inhibited transmission of small fibre impulses in the dorsal horn.

1.1.3 **Gate-control theory**

The gate-control theory was effectively a synthesis of the strongest elements of all these main theories. It recognized the specificity of peripheral pain systems, central summation, and input modulation via larger sensory fibres and psychological influences. The gate-control theory proposed a spinal gating mechanism in the dorsal horn that was influenced by the relative amounts of activity in large and small fibres and by descending controls from the brain. Thus, pain is a complex experience of somatic mechanisms and psychological influences (affective and cognitive) and, as such, is always subjective in nature.

1.1.4 **Current model**

Increasing neuroscience evidence suggests that the nervous system is capable of substantial plasticity. This is the ordered alteration of structure or function due to development, experience, or injury. Central neurons have the capacity to change their responsiveness in spatial, temporal, and amplitude aspects to a given stimulus, especially if the stimulus is chronic. This 'jungle of neurochemical anatomy' can undoubtedly account for this plastic nature but the exact mechanisms are still being elucidated. The plasticity theory is the most comprehensive pain model to date.

1.2 **Classification of pain**

1.2.1 **Physiological or pathological?**

Attempts at the classification of pain continue to evolve but, to date, all generally reflect the underlying pathophysiological mechanisms that are thought to *initiate* the pain. Although this classification of pain is simplistic, it affords a working paradigm in the pain clinic and is generally accepted by practitioners.

Pain classifications generally propose that pain is either physiological (normal) or pathological (abnormal), although there is no universally accepted system. Physiological pain results from the activation of peripheral nociceptive afferents by noxious (potentially harmful) stimuli assuming baseline sensitivity of the sensory system and serves to warn of impending tissue injury. Here, pain is a normal experience that is essential to the survival of the individual though a well argued editorial suggests that this concept may be flawed (see Nash 2005).

Pathological pain is distinguished by a change in baseline sensitivity of the nervous system and occurs after injury. This serves to protect the individual from further injury while healing occurs, an adaptive response. Pathological pain is termed 'maladaptive' when the sensitivity of the sensory system does not return to normal after tissue healing. Nociceptive pain is pain that occurs due to normal activation of the nociceptive system either by impending tissue injury or ongoing tissue destruction or inflammation.

This model has been developed further into a three-level classification which incorporates firstly the mechanism (nociceptive or neuropathic), then the context (physiological or pathological), and finally the location (somatic, e.g. bone; or visceral, e.g. bowel) (Fig. 1.1).

1.2.2 Mechanism based

Recently, a more fundamental mechanism-based classification of pain has been proposed. In this system, pain symptoms, mechanisms, and syndromes form a new hierarchy which does not involve traditional dichotomies such as malignant/non-malignant or acute/chronic. Two broad pain categories are identified – tissue injury pain (inflammatory) or nervous system injury pain – both of which encompass a number of universal mechanisms.

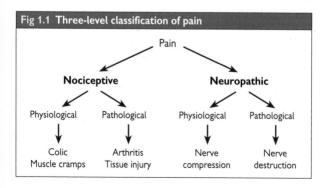

Fig 1.1 Three-level classification of pain

Pain

Nociceptive | Neuropathic

Physiological | Pathological | Physiological | Pathological

Colic
Muscle cramps | Arthritis
Tissue injury | Nerve
compression | Nerve
destruction

1.3 **History of neuropathic pain**

Dysfunction of the nervous system as a cause of chronic pain had been recognised by Galen in the second century AD, but it was after the Middle Ages that more consistent reports have been found. The increasing use of guns in wars from the seventeenth century onwards accounted for a great deal of traumatic nerve injury suffered by those that survived such injuries. Another feature of military life that began around this time was the recording and treatment of injuries by medical and nursing personnel accompanying the army.

Several of these accounts match contemporary descriptions of neuropathic pain. Dr Weir-Mitchell famously published his descriptions of pain associated with peripheral nerve injuries in Unionist soldiers of the American Civil War in 1864 and coined the term 'causalgia'. Ideas as to the mechanisms of pain that resulted from neural injury surfaced early in the twentieth century. However, steady growth of neuropathic pain research did not occur until the late 1970s when the special nature of neuropathic pain had been recognized and distinct terminology had emerged.

1.4 **Current taxonomy**

1.4.1 **Neuropathic pain definitions**

Neuropathy is defined as the disturbance of function or pathological change in a nerve. Hence the definition for neuropathic pain by the International Association for the Study of Pain (IASP) is 'pain initiated or caused by a primary lesion or dysfunction of the nervous system'. Neuropathic pain is best thought of as an *abnormal* activation of pain pathways and can occur as a result of injury or dysfunction to peripheral nerves and posterior roots (peripheral neuropathic pain) and spinal cord and brain (central pain). Table 1.1 contains examples of clinical neuropathic pains.

Despite 'neuropathic pain' being the preferred term, there has been some confusion over the terminology of this pain-generating mechanism. Some authors prefer the term 'neurogenic pain' while others prefer 'deafferentation pain' (this denotes complete nerve destruction with loss of afferent input beyond this point). Both are used as umbrella terms for peripheral neuropathic pain and central neuropathic pain.

1.4.2 **Types of neuropathic pain**

The distinction between physiological and pathological neuropathic pain has been made. The former includes nerve compression pain

Table 1.1 Examples of neuropathic pain		
Origin of pain	**Structure**	**Example**
Peripheral nervous system	Nerve	Neuroma
		Diabetic neuropathy
		Phantom limb pain
		Trigeminal neuralgia
		Lumbosacral plexopathy
	Dorsal root	Post-herpetic neuralgia
		Brachial plexus avulsion
Central nervous system	Spinal cord	Spinal cord injury
		Spinal cord ischaemia
	Brain	Wallenberg's syndrome
		Multiple sclerosis

which produces a *reversible* dysfunction of the nerve provided the compression is transient. Clinically, the symptoms of nerve compression are not easy to distinguish from nerve destruction. A further distinction is made with pseudoneuropathic pain in which patients display typical symptoms and signs of neuropathic pain but have no demonstrable nerve dysfunction on rigorous laboratory and neurological testing. It is thought to have a psychogenic origin but its existence remains subject to debate.

1.4.3 Role of autonomic system

Until recently, pain associated with autonomic dysfunction was considered separately from neuropathic pain. It has now been included in this category on the grounds that it represents a dysfunction of regional sympathetic nerves and the clinical features are similar to those of other neuropathic pains. Confusion over the classification of autonomic dysfunction remains. Some authors divide pain associated with autonomic dysfunction into sympathetically maintained pain (SMP) or sympathetically independent pain (SIP) according to whether the patient's pain improves or not after sympathetic blockade, though this has been shown to be an unreliable test.

Sympathetic pain has undergone several redefinitions including CPSMV (Chronic Pain associated with various combinations of positive and negative Sensory, Motor and Vasomotor phenomena). In the last 10 years it has come to be known as Complex Regional Pain Syndrome (see Chapter 7). The change in definition reflects the unpredictable contribution of autonomic dysfunction to neuropathic pain and the uncertainty over causal mechanisms.

1.5 Future definition of neuropathic pain

Currently, the very definition of neuropathic pain is hotly debated. Some pain clinicians argue for a narrow definition of nerve dysfunction. This neurologically based definition proposes that demonstrable nerve injury or damage (i.e. pathological neuropathic pain) is the only criteria for neuropathic pain or 'hypersensitivity pain disorder'. Others argue for a broader definition where dysfunction alone (i.e. presence of abnormal activity), but not necessarily identifiable or known nerve damage, should be included within the criteria for neuropathic pain.

This effectively means that some cases of complex regional pain syndrome (CRPS), fibromyalgia, and even irritable bowel syndrome fall within this broader umbrella of neuropathic pain. An analogy has been made with Parkinson's disease, which was originally known as a dysfunction of the extrapyramidal motor system before the exact mechanism was elucidated. Now, of course, it is known that atrophy of dopaminergic neurons in the substantia nigra results in the clinical manifestations of Parkinson's disease. A sensible view expressed in the literature is that more effort should be applied to understanding the mechanisms of pains such as CRPS, rather than argue about their inclusion as types of neuropathic pain.

Key references

Backonja, M.M. (2003). Defining neuropathic pain. *Anesth. Analg.*, **97**, 785–90.

Bennett, G.J. (2003). Neuropathic pain: a crisis of definition? *Anesth. Analg.*, **97**, 619–20.

Melzack, R. and Wall, P.D. (1965). Pain mechanisms: a new theory. *Science*, **150**, 971–9.

Merskey, H. and Bogduk, N. (1994). *Classification of chronic pain: descriptions of chronic pain syndromes and definitions of pain terms* (2nd edn). IASP Press, Seattle.

Nash, T. (2005). 'What use is pain?' *British Journal of Anaesthesia*, **94**(2), 146–149.

Woolf, C.J., Bennett, G.J., Doherty, M., Dubner, R., Kidd, B., Koltzenburg, M., et al. (1998). Towards a mechanism-based classification of pain? *Pain*, **77**, 227–9.

Chapter 2

Pathophysiology of neuropathic pain

Catherine E. Urch

> **Key points**
>
> - Noxious stimuli are coded and transmitted via Aδ and C primary afferent neurons in the periphery to the dorsal horn of the spinal cord.
> - In the dorsal horn, transmission of noxious stimuli involves the neurotransmitters glutamate and substance P, but input can be inhibited or amplified by other influences.
> - Damage to peripheral nerves can result in reduced firing thresholds, ectopic discharges, and cross-talk (activation of adjacent normal nerves).
> - Abnormal peripheral input or direct damage to the central nervous system leads to hyperexcitability and loss of inhibition.
> - Neuropathic pain states can impact on control of descending inhibitory pathways from higher brain centres.

Pain arising after nerve injury or damage is a challenge to both clinicians and scientists. In other areas of nerve damage, sensory loss is expected, such as with vision. However, the question is when neuronal damage is inflicted on nociceptive neurons, why is there both loss, in the form of numbness, and abnormal gains in the form of pain and hyperalgesia?

2.1 Normal transmission

2.1.1 Activation in the periphery

Pain is normally elicited only when a noxious (potentially harmful) stimulus activates the high-threshold peripheral nociceptors. The peripheral nervous system is differentiated into Aβ fibres, which are activated by non-noxious (non-harmful) stimuli; and Aδ and C primary afferent fibres, which specifically code for noxious stimuli, such as heat, chemical, pressure, and inflammation. These stimuli activate specific receptors on the neuron (such as acid-sensing receptors [ASIC] and prostaglandin receptors), which in turn allow the neuron to depolarize by an influx of positive ions, usually sodium and calcium. Once a threshold is reached the neuron continues to carry the depolarization up to its cell body, the dorsal root ganglion (DRG), and the dorsal horn within the spinal cord.

2.1.2 Activity in the central nervous system

Once in the spinal cord the neuron releases transmitters, such as glutamate and substance P, which travel across the synapse to the post-synaptic neurons and glial cells. The neurons can be inhibitory (gamma amino butyric acid [GABA]-ergic) or excitatory inter-neurons, whilst the glial cells play an active role in removing and releasing neurotransmitters. The dorsal horn can modulate the input of the primary afferent neuron to allow magnification (excitation, with 'wind-up') or reduction (inhibition). The net result is passed via the ascending tracts (such as spinothalamic, parabrachial) to the higher brain centres involved in the coding, modulating, and the experience of pain. The brain in turn sends excitatory and inhibitory signals back to the dorsal horn via the descending pathways, which in turn further modulate the output.

2.2 Peripheral changes following damage

Neuropathic pain is characterized by spontaneous pain (stimulus-independent), hyperalgesia (increased pain to a given noxious stimulus), and allodynia (pain arising from non-noxious stimuli). Some of these clinical characteristics may be explained by the alterations that occur within the peripheral nerves following damage.

2.2.1 Reduced thresholds

If the milieu surrounding a peripheral neuron is altered, or the nerve is compressed or damaged, the receptors that normally transduce stimuli at certain intensities can be activated at lower intensities. For example, with cell damage, death, or inflammation, the pH can be reduced and thus activate the ASIC channels, or Adenosine Tri-Phosphate (ATP) receptors (P_2X_3). This in turn can lead to the neuron being always partially or totally depolarized. In the former, it wouldn't take much further activation, say by a prostaglandin or bradykinin receptor activation, to make the neuron fire. The normally high-threshold neuron will now be activated with a lower threshold stimulus, which is seen in hyperalgesia.

2.2.2 Altered transmission

Normal transmission relies on ordered sequential functioning of sodium and calcium channels, allowing depolarization to occur in a specific place and time. In damaged neurons, perhaps caused by transection following surgery or amputation, the severed neuron responds to the loss of its distal portion by trying to regrow ('sprouting'), forming a neuroma which is a whorl of neuronal tissue with or without myelin. Neurons also develop abnormal accumulations of sodium and calcium channels which are not only abnormal in density (increased), but also undergo a change in character and activation properties.

There are nine different sodium channels currently identified which possess different characteristics with respect to what voltage they open at, how long they stay open, how quickly they close (inactivate), and the refractory time before reopening. The distribution of sodium channels alters with development, type of neuron, and in response to damage. For example, it has been shown that a fetal sodium channel, $Na_v1.3$, is up-regulated following neuropathy, $Na_v1.8$ is located on small-diameter primary afferents (Aδ and C fibres), whilst $Na_v1.7$ is on all size fibres. Work suggests that the differential expression and accumulation of sodium channels is responsible for spontaneous discharges in damaged neurons (called ectopic discharges), which may be perceived as spontaneous pain. Normally, nerve impulses are generated at sensory terminals. In pathological states, impulses may arise from the damaged part of the axon and propagate toward both the central nervous system and the periphery. Such ectopic discharges may also arise from local patches of demyelination, neuroma, and the dorsal root ganglion.

Likewise, the calcium channels belong to a large family, and are differentially located depending on neuronal type and damage. All calcium channels contain a sub-unit $\alpha_2\delta$, which is an important therapeutic target for gabapentin. Remodelling of other membrane channels is important, such as potassium channels, if not as well characterized (Fig. 2.1).

2.2.3 Other peripheral changes

The chaotic depolarization and transmission affects events:

- within the neuron – such as altered retrograde translation of nerve growth factor
- within the dorsal root ganglion – activation of *c-fos* and other genes, with the result of altered receptor and secondary messenger translation
- between neurons
- within the dorsal horn.

In the periphery, the abnormal neuronal sprouting can lead to an enlargement of the receptive field (area of body) that feeds the abnormal pain transmission. These nerve endings also 'cross-talk' to other non-damaged nerves, in turn altering the normal nerves to become abnormal and chaotic. Likewise, the damaged neuron itself engages in 'ephatic' cross-talk to non-damaged neurons within its bundle. This cross-talk causes a synchronous depolarization and

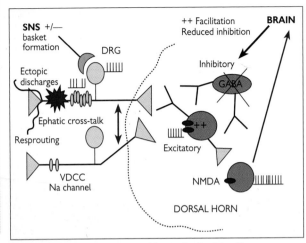

Figure 2.1 A diagrammatic summary of the peripheral and dorsal horn
pro-excitatory changes following a peripheral nerve injury. In the periphery, there is
an increase in density and activity of sodium (Na) and voltage-dependent calcium
channels (VDCC), leading to ectopic discharge. There is also ephatic cross-talk
between damaged and undamaged neurons and sprouting of the damaged neuron,
all leading to an increase in receptive field size. In some cases the sympathetic
nervous system (SNS) may form aberrant sprouting, leading to basket formation
around abnormal dorsal root ganglion (DRG). The dorsal horn is pro-excitatory,
as illustrated by an increasing number of action potentials with each inter-neuron.
The excitation is in part driven by the activation of NMDA receptors, amongst
others, and the overall reduction of inhibition, either intrinsic – GABA-ergic loss,
inhibited opioid receptors – or extrinsic – reduced descending inhibition and
increased descending facilitation.

perpetuates the pathological characteristics onto otherwise normal
non-damaged neurons.

2.3 Alterations within the dorsal horn

2.3.1 Peripheral inputs

The dorsal horn is a central point of modulation of normal pain
signals, and is also vital to the onward transmission of the abnormal
and chaotic inputs from damaged (and adjacent) non-damaged
neurons. The Aδ and C fibres terminate predominantly in the superficial layers (lamina I and II) of the dorsal horn, also Aδ in lamina V,
and the non-noxious Aβ fibres terminate in lamina III. Work of some
years ago suggested that there was abnormal resprouting of Aβ
fibres into lamina II, thus allowing non-painful thresholds to be trans-
lated in the dorsal horn as pain. This would have accounted nicely for
the symptom of allodynia. This theory, whilst widely quoted and

beguiling in its neatness, has in many elements been disproved and dorsal horn neuronal reorganization should be viewed as contentious. It appears that C fibres take on characteristics of, and express receptors that are normally confined to, low-threshold Aβ fibres.

2.3.2 Role of NMDA receptors

Within the dorsal horn the abnormal primary afferent inputs result in areas of 'silence' (with no input) and areas of chaotic over-activity. The increased release of neurotransmitters allows the prolonged depolarization of the post-synaptic neurons, and the activation of the N-methyl D-aspartate (NMDA) receptor. This receptor is important, as it usually remains closed by magnesium ion block until both the cell is depolarized and there continues to be glutamate (and glycine) binding to the receptor (Fig. 2.2; see also Chapter 11). Once these multiple events occur, the receptor opens and allows a flood of calcium and sodium into the cell. The effect is one of massive excitation within the neuron, known as 'wind-up', a greatly increased response to a given stimuli. Increase of calcium within the cell not only activates and depolarizes it, but also sets in train a series of events that modifies receptors (either more open or more closed), activates secondary messenger pathways, alters gene expression, increases the production of excitatory gases such as nitric oxide, and other effects. The overall effect is one of neuronal excitation.

13

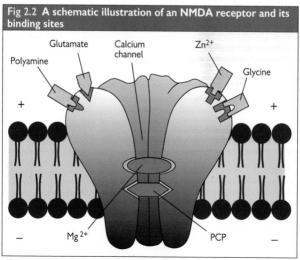

Fig 2.2 A schematic illustration of an NMDA receptor and its binding sites

Polyamine · Glutamate · Calcium channel · Zn²⁺ · Glycine · + · + · − · Mg²⁺ · PCP · −

Figure 2.2 reproduced with permission from Neil Camson

Foundations of Physiological Psychology, 6e Published by Allyn and Bacon, Boston, MA. Copyright © 2004 by Peason Education.

In addition it appears that there is an overall reduction in the inhibition within the dorsal horn, either by loss or down-regulation of GABA-ergic neurons, or loss of active intrinsic opioid receptors, combined with reduction in descending inhibitory pathways (see Fig. 2.1).

2.4 Alterations centrally

2.4.1 Descending pathways

Serotonergic pathways appear to be central in the descending facilitatory pathway. From lamina I of the dorsal horn, the parabrachial pathway ascends to the brainstem (hypothalamus, perception). The signals are modulated and transmitted to the peri-aquaductal grey (PAG) and rostro-ventral medulla (RVM) from where the descending system commences and terminates back within the spinal cord. It has been shown that the attention/distraction centre of the PAG is aberrant in humans with chronic pain, who could not activate descending inhibition. It must be remembered that whilst the ascending spinothalamic pathways retain a strict location mapping, the parabrachial and descending systems are diffuse and lack location map (Fig. 2.3).

2.4.2 Control of descending pathways

The peripheral and dorsal horn alterations have been investigated extensively for decades in animal models. The areas are readily accessible and much has been elucidated about the pathophysiological state that follows neuropathic injury, which has been largely confirmed in human studies.

The more central areas within the brain have remained a black box for some time. However, over the last decade sophisticated animal work within the RVM and PAG have revealed a complex web of interconnecting neurons, with specific 'on', 'off', and 'neutral' cells which are central in controlling descending pathways back to the dorsal horn. These areas in turn have projections to and from multiple other areas such as the sensory cortex and hypothalamus. The recent refinement of functional magnetic resonance imaging (fMRI) and positron emission tomography (PET) imaging has allowed a more clinically based approach to understanding the complex interconnections and plasticity within the brain following neuropathic injury (Fig. 2.3).

2.4.3 Higher brain centres

Extensive modulation, excitation, and abnormal changes that occur in primary afferents and the dorsal horn continue throughout the higher pain centres, in particular the RVM, PAG, thalamus, primary somatosensory cortex (S1 and S2), and anterior cingulate cortex. Recent fMRI work has suggested that distinct regions of the brain are activated with noxious

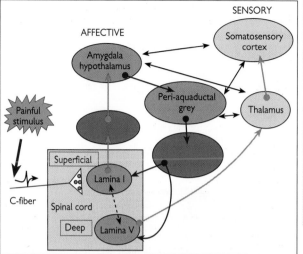

Figure 2.3 A summary of some of the interactions between the peripheral neurons, dorsal horn, and higher centres in the brain. As illustrated, the noxious coding Aδ and C fibres terminate in the superficial (lamina I /II) and deep (lamina V) dorsal horn. However, the ascending pathways are distinct. The predominant pathway to the sensory cortex, coding for intensity and location of the stimulus, is via the spinothalamic tract, whilst the parabrachial pathway is predominately responsible for linking lamina I with the hypothalamus and amygdala. This codes for the affective and recall component of pain perception, which is neither location nor intensity specific. All the centres in the brain have large projections between them, each allowing extensive modulation of the initial input. The descending pathways arise within the peri-aquadactal grey and rostro-ventral medulla, and translate inhibitory and facilitatory inputs back to the dorsal horn. The motor response generated from the cortex is not displayed.

stimuli, pain, anticipation, recall, and emotion, and are altered in states of chronic pain. Also fMRI has allowed the study of clinical pain states and has shown extensive plasticity, remapping, and excitation, which alter pre- and post-pain control. For example, in complex regional pain syndrome (CRPS; see Chapter 7) the areas that map body location in the cortex showed a reduction in the space between them, this reverted to normal spacing when the pain had been controlled.

2.5 Interpreting pathophysiology

The more important and well-documented changes that occur following nerve damage have been reviewed and outlined. Neuropathic pain is clearly a pathological state peripherally, within the dorsal horn and higher central structures. Neuropathy is not, however, one uniform state. Some of the alterations (such as NMDA activation) probably occur in all states, others (such as sympathetic nervous system [SNS] aberrant basket formation) do not. It is appealing to think that a mechanism-based approach to the diagnosis and treatment of neuropathic pain may be here soon, however caution should be used in trying to dissect a complex, inter-dependent, plastic state into a few measurable receptors.

Key references

Carpenter, K.J. and Dickenson, A.H. (2002). Molecular aspects of pain research. *Pharmacogenomics J.*, **2**, 87–95.

Cervero, F. and Laird, J.M. (2004). Understanding the signalling and transmission of visceral nociceptive events. *J. Neurobiol.*, **61**, 45–54.

Suzuki, R. and Dickenson, A.H. (2000). Neuropathic pain: nerves bursting with excitement. *Neuroreport*, **11**, R17–21.

Suzuki, R., Rygh, L.J., and Dickenson, A.H. (2004). Bad news from the brain: descending 5-HT pathways that control spinal pain processing. *Trends Pharmacol. Sci.*, **25**, 613–17.

Tracey, I. (2005). Functional connectivity and pain: how effectively connected is your brain? *Pain*, **116**, 173–4.

Tsuda, M., Inoue, K., and Salter, M.W. (2005). Neuropathic pain and spinal microglia: a big problem from molecules in 'small' glia. *Trends Neurosci.*, **28**, 101–7.

Woolf, C.J. and Mannion, R.J. (1999). Neuropathic pain: aetiology, symptoms, mechanisms and management. *Lancet*, **353**, 1959–64.

Chapter 3

Epidemiology

Blair H. Smith and Nicola Torrance

Key points

- Lack of agreed definitions and diagnostic criteria for neuropathic pain hamper epidemiological studies.
- Neuropathic pain is likely to become more common in future because of ageing populations and improved recognition.
- Neuropathic pain probably affects around 8% of UK adults, around 24% or more of patients with long-standing diabetes, and around 20% of those who have had shingles.
- Patients with neuropathic pain are more likely to have greater pain intensity, be older, of female gender, and of lower socio-economic status than those with other types of pain.
- Compared with other forms of chronic pain, neuropathic pain leads to greater detrimental impact on activities of daily living and lower health-related quality of life scores.

3.1 Introduction

3.1.1 Role of epidemiology

The experience of neuropathic pain is generally more distressing than that of other forms of pain, and it can be a significant challenge for physicians to treat or control it. Epidemiology is one important discipline in the struggle to improve this situation. Epidemiology is 'the study of the distribution and determinants of health-related states ... and the application of this study to the control of health problems'. It is the latter part of this definition that makes epidemiology an important clinical discipline, particularly for neuropathic pain.

3.1.2 Challenges in neuropathic pain

Keys to epidemiological study include an agreed case definition and a standardized method of case identification or ascertainment.

Unfortunately neither of these currently exists for neuropathic pain. The International Association for the Study of Pain defines it as pain 'initiated or caused by a primary lesion or dysfunction in the nervous system'. This pathophysiological definition has limited practical value for either clinical or epidemiological classification. The range of possible causes of neuropathic pain is wide and diverse, and arguments exist against classification as a single global entity.

However, others argue, and evidence suggests, that there are enough similarities between all causes of neuropathic pain in the mechanisms generating the pain, the symptoms experienced, the signs elicited, and the impact on quality of life to merit detailed universal study. Most importantly, perhaps, there are similarities in the response to treatment, distinct from other types of pain. Pharmacologically, there is good evidence for different types of neuropathic pain to be considered together, irrespective of aetiology.

A uniform approach to describing the epidemiology of neuropathic pain will therefore provide an understanding of the scale of the problem throughout the community (and not simply those attending the pain clinic), evidence for the development of strategies for treatment or prevention, and will allow the targeting of medical and educational resources. Good epidemiological research can also provide the basis for the design of clinical trials, including adequate power calculations.

3.2 Epidemiology of neuropathic pain as a single entity

3.2.1 Historical estimates

In 1991, a British paper suggested that the prevalence of neuropathic pain in the UK general population was probably about 1%, though this was based on estimates rather than direct evidence. A similar, though more detailed, approach in the USA derived a broadly similar estimate in 1997. However, these global calculations are likely to be inaccurate, based as they are on a series of estimates of variable validity. They cannot take into consideration pain with neuropathic characteristics that has not been formally classified with one of the traditionally recognized clinical diagnoses or causes, leading to possible underestimates. On the other hand, they may count individuals who have more than one relevant diagnosis twice, leading to possible overestimates.

3.2.2 The need for case definition instruments

There are no agreed, standardized guidelines that allow clinicians to classify pain type (neuropathic or nociceptive) without controversy. Equally, there are no case definition instruments that can do the same for epidemiological research. This is partly because the development of these would have to be based on agreed clinical standards, but also partly because of the current debate, which suggests that many (or even most) pain diagnoses comprise a mixture of neuropathic and nociceptive mechanisms (see Chapter 4). Neuropathic pain is not necessarily a binary phenomenon, i.e. present or absent, but may be a spectrum; neuropathic mechanisms may contribute a greater or lesser component to the overall aetiology of an individual's pain.

Epidemiological study is therefore most profitably aimed at identifying pain of predominantly neuropathic origin, as this is where specific therapy should be targeted. Instruments have been developed based on this principle, including the Douleur Neuropathique 4 (DN4) and the Leeds Assessment of Neuropathic Symptoms and Signs, which now includes a self-complete version, the S-LANSS (see Chapter 4 and Appendix 2). The latter now allows an evidence-based estimate of the population prevalence of pain of predominantly neuropathic origin (POPNO).

3.2.3 Current estimates

A recent UK study used the S-LANSS in a postal survey of 6000 adults randomly selected from general practices. Among the responders, the study found that the population prevalence of chronic pain of predominantly neuropathic origin was 8.2% in adults. This represented 17% of those with chronic pain, included a range of pain diagnoses, and was commoner among women, older respondents, and those with poorer indices of socio-economic status. The reporting of neuropathic pain was also associated with greater pain severity and health-seeking behaviours. Neuropathic pain in the community therefore seems to be more common than previously estimated.

The prevalence of neuropathic pain can be expected to increase in the future as the population ages. As well as the association with age found in the above study, a number of causes of neuropathic pain are found to be more common in the elderly, including herpes zoster and diabetic neuropathy. Patients with chronic diseases that are associated with neuropathic pain – for example, cancer, HIV, and diabetes – are also surviving longer due to improved medical care.

3.3 Epidemiology of individual neuropathic pain syndromes

3.3.1 Post-herpetic neuralgia and painful diabetic neuropathy

Depending upon where the nerve lesion or dysfunction is located, neuropathic pain may be defined as peripheral or central (Box 3.1). It was this type of classification that led to the USA estimate of prevalence described above. The epidemiology of many of these individual diagnoses has been researched to greater or lesser extent, including

> **Box 3.1 Some common causes of neuropathic pain**
>
> **Peripheral nerve lesion or dysfunction**
> - Painful diabetic neuropathy
> - Post-herpetic neuralgia
> - Post-surgical pain (including post-mastectomy and phantom limb pain)
> - Complex regional pain syndrome
> - Trigeminal neuralgia
> - Chemotherapy-induced neuropathy
> - Neuropathy secondary to tumour infiltration
>
> **Central nerve lesion or dysfunction**
> - Central post-stroke pain
> - Multiple sclerosis pain
> - Spinal cord injury pain

the two commonest and best understood: painful diabetic neuropathy (PDN) and post-herpetic neuralgia (PHN).

Peripheral neuropathy affects perhaps a third of individuals with diabetes mellitus, though this is not always associated with pain. Depending upon the definition and severity of pain, and the type of diabetes, neuropathic pain has been found to affect between 11% and 24% of people with diabetes. The precise mechanism of pain remains unclear; so do the associations with duration and severity of diabetes, or its control, though these are all probably important. Painful diabetic neuropathy is commoner in older age groups.

The lifetime prevalence of herpes zoster infection has been estimated to be 10% to 20% in the general population and as high as 50% of a cohort living to age 85 years. Of these people, between 15% and 22% have been found to develop chronic pain at the site of the shingles rash: post-herpetic neuralgia. Like PDN, PHN is commoner in older people. Other risk factors include female gender, severity of shingles and associated acute pain, and psychosocial factors including distress and living alone.

3.3.2 **Other neuropathic pain conditions**

Examples of other chronic pain conditions with neuropathic mechanisms for which we have detailed epidemiological information include:

- post-surgical pain
- phantom limb pain
- central post-stroke pain
- temperomandibular disorder pain
- cancer pain.

Note that these conditions are not exclusively neuropathic pain conditions. Some include a range of pain mechanisms, and others are caused by mixed nociceptive and neuropathic mechanisms. Most individuals with these conditions will have pain somewhere on the spectrum described above. A wide range of prevalence figures and risk factors is available for each of these conditions, depending on the precise definition of the condition and of pain in the studies conducted. Readers are referred to a review published by the International Association for the Study of Pain (IASP) or the detailed scientific literature available for more information.

3.3.3 Risk factors and natural history

Information on the long-term natural history of neuropathic pain is scant. However, from the evidence that does exist, it seems that the outlook is generally poor, with no or little change in symptoms found in follow-up studies. Therefore, once chronic neuropathic pain is established, it seems to be permanent in most cases. Epidemiological study should therefore consider risk factors for its development, with a view to its prevention or limitation.

Common risk factors for neuropathic pain conditions found throughout the literature include older age, female gender, and indices of deprivation or relatively low socio-economic status. These are not modifiable, at least not by a physician, and are therefore mostly of academic or political interest, though it is worth noting the parallels with other chronic pain and non-pain conditions.

Of greater clinical interest, perhaps, are the psychosocial risk factors (such as the association between distress and PHN), as well as some clinical factors specific for each condition. These may be amenable to intervention, and therefore prevention or limitation of neuropathic pain. Research is still required in this area, but several findings show promise. For example, less intense post-mastectomy pain in the acute phase after surgery may be associated with reduced chronic neuropathic pain. Prevention should therefore focus on the immediate post-operative phase, though this requires detailed confirmation. Counselling or other psychological interventions aimed at the reduction of distress might also be effective in reducing chronic pain after surgery or amputation. Again, confirmation is required through clinical trials, and these are active or planned in several locations.

3.4 Impact of neuropathic pain

3.4.1 Quality-of-life measures

Although there is a lack of general population research in this area, studies consistently find that individuals with neuropathic pain conditions have poorer health than those without in every health dimension measured: physical, psychological, and social. They also have more severe, unpleasant pain than those with other types of chronic pain. This research confirms clinical impressions, and tells us that these patients have greater disruption of daily activity, poorer sleep and quality of life, and poorer mental health than they would if their pain could be adequately treated. This could be said of any chronic pain, but seems to be particularly true for neuropathic pain.

3.4.2 Measuring improvement

The Neuropathic Pain Scale (NPS; see Chapter 4) was developed to measure specific characteristics of the experience of chronic pain. It includes sub-scales measuring the pain's intensity, heat, sharpness, hypersensitivity, and unpleasantness, all of which score higher among people with neuropathic pain than with other pain types. The fact that these sub-scales are sensitive to change, and their scores improve with treatment (such as gabapentin or lidocaine patches), confirms the benefits of intervention. Several studies have also shown improvements in measures of general physical, psychological, and social well-being as secondary outcomes of interventions for neuropathic pain. Further research is required in the general population to establish baseline and natural history data.

3.5 Further epidemiological research

3.5.1 Need for consensus on definitions

Further advances in the epidemiological understanding of neuropathic pain are hampered by the absence of agreed detailed definitions and diagnostic criteria for classifying neuropathic pain. If and when these are established, standard instruments can be developed for case identification and ascertainment in research. Until then, our information must continue to be drawn from study of specific conditions with neuropathic mechanisms of pain (such as PDN), or from pragmatic approximations (such as 'pain of predominantly neuropathic origin'). To a certain extent the current debate about the mechanisms and binary nature of neuropathic pain will need to be resolved before these gold standards can be designed and accepted widely. However, this must not hamper clinical progress unduly.

3.5.2 Improving prevention and management strategies

The important outcome of epidemiological research in neuropathic pain, as with all other conditions, is the further development of prevention and management strategies. If these are successful, a great deal of suffering will be relieved.

Existing epidemiological tools such as the S-LANSS and DN4 have an important place, but need further validation, particularly in general population settings. This will allow large-scale population-based research, and a clearer understanding of the aetiology, incidence, risk factors, and natural history associated with chronic neuropathic pain.

This information is crucial in the design of prevention strategies, or of interventions designed to minimize disability and maximize capacity. It is also important in the design of the clinical trials to which the epidemiological research must all lead, including targeting interventions, identifying important outcome measures, and powering studies with appropriate sample sizes. A particularly exciting possibility is the study of genetic mechanisms in the development of neuropathic pain, and there are several large population studies underway internationally that may eventually allow this.

Key references

Bowsher, D. (1991). Neurogenic pain syndromes and their management. *Br. Med. Bull.*, **47**, 644–66.

Bowsher, D. (1999). The lifetime occurrence of herpes zoster and prevalence of postherpetic neuralgia: a retrospective survey in an elderly population. *Eur. J. Pain*, **3**, 335–42.

Crombie, I.K., Croft, P.R., Linton, S.J., LeResche, L., and Von Korff, M. (ed.) (1999). *Epidemiology of pain*. IASP Press, Seattle.

Dworkin, R.H. (2002). An overview of neuropathic pain: syndromes, symptoms, signs, and several mechanisms. *Clin. J. Pain*, **18**, 343–9.

Dworkin, R.H. and Schmader, K.E. (2001). The epidemiology and natural history of herpes zoster and postherpetic neuralgia. In: C.P.N. Watson (ed.) *Herpes zoster and postherpetic neuralgia* (2nd edn), pp. 39–65. Elsevier, Amsterdam.

Hansson, P.T. and Dickenson, A.H. (2005). Pharmacological treatment of peripheral neuropathic pain conditions on shared commonalities despite multiple etiologies. *Pain*, **113**, 251–4.

Schmader, K.E. (2002). Epidemiology and impact on quality of life of postherpetic neuralgia and painful diabetic neuropathy. *Clin. J. Pain*, **18**, 350–4.

Torrance, N., Smith, B.H., Bennett, M., and Lee, A.J. (2006). The epidemiology of chronic pain of predominantly neuropathic origin. Results from a general population study. *J. Pain*, **7**(4), 281–289.

Chapter 4

Diagnosing neuropathic pain in clinical practice

Michael I. Bennett

Key points

- Neuropathic pain can be difficult to identify because it is subjective, evidence of neuropathy does not always imply neuropathic pain, and multiple pathological mechanisms are variously expressed, some of which overlap with nociceptive pain.
- Common symptoms are spontaneous pains (those that arise without detectable stimulation) and evoked pains (abnormal responses to stimulation).
- Common signs are allodynia, hyperalgesia, hyperpathia, autonomic dysfunction, and sensory loss.
- Verbal pain description has an important role in identifying neuropathic pain and scales such as the LANSS and NPS are standardized approaches.
- An emerging concept is that pain can be more or less neuropathic; clinicians should ask themselves, 'what is the dominance of neuropathic mechanisms in this pain state?'

4.1 Difficulties in identifying neuropathic pain

4.1.1 Pain is subjective

Identifying neuropathic pain in clinical practice is not easy. The sensation of pain itself cannot be objectively measured and there remain no agreed diagnostic criteria for neuropathic pain. Although many pain questionnaires exist and certain behaviours have been identified that are associated with pain states, they are only subjective and corroborative measures, respectively.

4.1.2 **Neuropathy does not equal pain**

The distinction between nociceptive and neuropathic pain mechanisms is often a difficult clinical exercise. The underlying pathophysiological mechanisms that result in chronic pain can only be inferred. This inference is based primarily on verbal description supported by examination and investigations. This amounts to a diagnostic probability rather than objective identification of a definitive mechanism.

Even if neuropathy can be identified objectively, it cannot be assumed that a causal relationship exists with the patient's pain; for example, painful osteoarthritis in the ankles of an elderly woman with age-related painless peripheral neuropathy. This exercise is further complicated when multiple possible causes exist in the presence of a progressive pathological process; for example, a middle-aged man with a Pancoast's lung cancer eroding his brachial plexus and surrounding soft tissue.

4.1.3 **Multiple mechanisms**

The term 'neuropathic pain' does not represent a single neural mechanism but is instead a unifying hypothesis of many variously expressed mechanisms (see Chapter 2). These can result in common clinical features such as spontaneous continuous and paroxysmal pains, and evoked pains. However, often the relationship between pain symptoms and nerve pathology complicates any attempt to understand these processes. For example, a common neural injury such as amputation can result in no pain in some patients to severe pain in others, with a spectrum of positive sensory phenomena, outlined below.

One reason for this is that different types of nerves respond differently to injury and this in turn is probably influenced by genetic predisposition, type of insult, and background psychological factors. In addition, it also includes how well the post-injury pain was controlled in the ensuing hours, days, and weeks in which tissue healing occurred. Neuropathic pain can become apparent immediately following injury or be delayed for several years, often 'ignited' by a second injury in the same area or one close by.

4.1.4 **Similarities with nociceptive pain**

The labelling of pain based on tissue injury or nerve injury mechanisms has been described as an oversimplification of complex processes that involve multiple interacting mechanisms evolving over time. In fact, at a neurophysiological level, there are many similarities between neuropathic and nociceptive pain in experimental models. Nevertheless, clinicians have to start somewhere because neuropathic pain mechanisms require additional analgesic approaches to those used for nociceptive pain. An outline of common clinical features in neuropathic pain is given below.

4.2 **Symptoms**

Classically, patients with neuropathic pain complain of spontaneous pains (those that arise without detectable stimulation) and evoked pains (abnormal responses to stimulation). Spontaneous pains can be continuous, steady, and ongoing or they can be paroxysmal, episodic, and intermittent.

Continuous pain is largely felt in cutaneous or deep tissues and less commonly from viscera. Cutaneous pain is often described in terms of dysaesthesias – 'burning, cutting, pricking, tingling, and stabbing' – whereas deep pains can be represented by 'cramping, aching, throbbing, and crushing'. Paroxysmal qualities are usually described in terms of 'shooting, stabbing, lancinating, or jabbing'. These features can be variously expressed ranging from absence in some to a full spectrum of descriptions in others. Overall, the intensity of neuropathic pain has been rated as greater than that of nociceptive pain.

4.3 **Signs**

4.3.1 **Range of phenomena**

The demonstration of nerve dysfunction is important corroborating evidence in the diagnosis of neuropathic pain. Nerve dysfunction in this context can be represented by sensory, motor, or autonomic dysfunction, though it is not always possible to attribute dysfunction to a discrete neurological lesion. In order to make sense of neuropathic signs, it is helpful to divide features of neuropathic pain into positive or negative phenomena (Fig. 4.1).

4.3.2 **Positive signs**

Positive phenomena in neuropathic pain are diverse and are a combination of evoked pains and sensations. They are all generally exaggerated responses to stimulation and can be grouped according to the type of abnormality found: qualitative, quantitative, temporal, or spatial.

Allodynia is a common feature and is defined as pain due to a stimulus which does not normally provoke pain. This represents a *qualitative* abnormality in that the stimulus and response are in different modes. Three types of neuropathic allodynia are reported based on the initiating stimulus: mechanical (tactile), thermal (warm and cold), and movement. Mechanical allodynia and thermal allodynia in neuropathic pain patients are disorders of cutaneous, rather than visceral, sensation. Mechanical allodynia can be induced by punctate stimuli such as a pin prick (static mechanical allodynia) or more commonly by stroking movements (dynamic mechanical allodynia).

Fig 4.1 Organizational chart representing clinical features of neuropathic pain

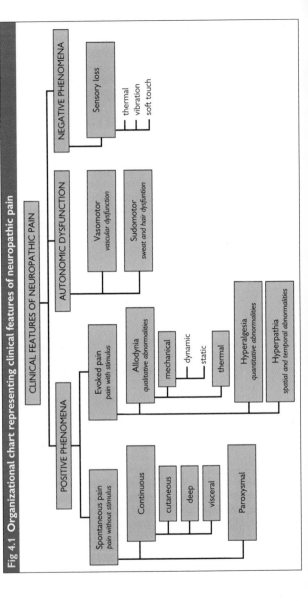

Hyperalgesia is a painful sensation of abnormal severity following a noxious stimulus and represents an exaggerated response to the same modality stimulus, a *quantitative* abnormality. Allodynia and hyperalgesia frequently coexist and in practice it can be difficult to differentiate the two. Both allodynia and hyperalgesia are reported to be pathognomonic of neuropathic pain but are in fact also associated with tissue damage and inflammation. However, when associated with chronic pain, these phenomena are most likely to represent a neuropathic mechanism. In contrast, allodynic sensations arising from innocuous stimulation of muscles, joints, and viscera (i.e. movement allodynia) are common following tissue injury but their existence in neuropathic pain is less well described.

Hyperpathia is characterized by *temporal* abnormalities such as increased reaction to a stimulus, particularly a repetitive stimulus, as well as an increased threshold. Prolonged painful after-sensations are also a feature. *Spatial* abnormalities such as dyslocalization (a stimulus in one area produces pain in another area) and radiation are other features of neuropathic pain.

Autonomic dysfunction can result in a wide range of vasomotor and sudomotor signs. Blood flow, skin temperature, and sweating can all be increased or decreased and vary within, as well as between, patients. Trophic changes are late signs of autonomic dysfunction.

4.3.3 Negative signs

Negative sensory manifestations can result in loss of light touch, vibration, pinprick, and thermal sensations. These sensations are mediated by larger myelinated Aβ fibres (light touch and vibration), Aδ (cold and pinprick sensations), and smaller unmyelinated C fibres (pain and warmth sensations). Objectively, impaired sensation to light touch and pinprick is used most frequently to determine nerve dysfunction, but clearly this will only identify dysfunction in Aβ and Aδ fibres. If the neuropathic process also involves motor nerves, muscle wasting with motor weakness will ensue.

4.4 Sensory testing

4.4.1 Role of clinical examination

A good working definition of neuropathic pain is 'pain occurring in an area of abnormal or absent sensation'. A more rigorous test is that neuropathic pain should only be diagnosed when the distribution of pain and the associated sensory abnormalities jointly, and in a clinical context, point to a neurological condition.

Examination of a patient with chronic pain should therefore focus on the location of pain and identifying any neurological abnormalities; in particular, detecting abnormal responses to a sensory stimulus. In practice, the commonest abnormalities are sensory loss (numbness at site of pain), allodynia, and hyperalgesia.

4.4.2 Bedside tests

There are several simple tests for detecting abnormal responses and all tests should compare the index site with a non-painful control site. Allodynia is best assessed by lightly brushing a piece of cotton wool over the site of pain. If pain is elicited (or sometimes unpleasant electrical feelings) in contrast to the control site, then allodynia is present (Fig. 4.2).

Hyper- and hypoalgesia are assessed by examining pinprick thresholds (PPT). A sharp wooden stick or, better still, a 23G needle mounted inside the barrel of a 2ml syringe (Fig. 4.3) is used to test the patient's ability to detect a sharp sensation at the site of pain compared with a control site. A raised PPT (patient cannot feel sharpness at site of pain) suggests hypoalgesia, a lowered PPT (patient feels exaggerated pain compared to control site) indicates hyperalgesia. Sometimes, standardized monofilaments are used to test detection thresholds and are commonly available as 1g or 10g (Fig. 4.4). By contrast, a 23G needle exerts about 0.5g. These have fixed tensions and so exert consistent pressure. Diabetic patients who fail to detect a 10g monofilament over their lower legs are at significant risk of neuropathic ulcers.

To test thermal sensations, the responses to a cold metal spoon and a warm examiner's finger can be compared at the site of pain and the control site. Inability to distinguish between cold and warm suggests abnormal C fibre function. Specially designed thermal rollers, set at specific and reliable temperatures, are available for more precise testing.

Fig 4.2 Testing for dynamic mechanical allodynia

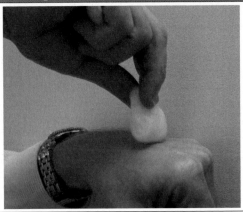

Fig 4.3 Testing for altered pin-prick threshold using 23G needle mounted inside 2ml syringe barrel

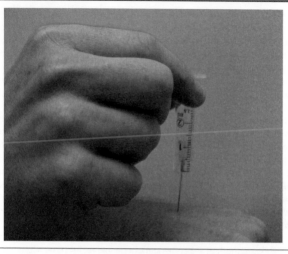

Fig 4.4 Testing for altered pin-prick threshold using monofilament

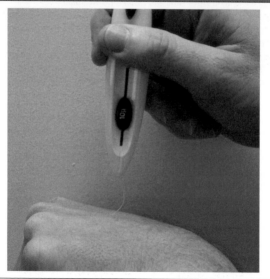

Any detected sensory abnormalities should be documented on a body-map in order to allow comparison on later retesting (Fig. 4.5).

4.4.3 Laboratory measurements

The demonstration and quantification of sensory dysfunction that accompanies pain is important in the diagnosis of neuropathic pain. This has proved challenging because pain is a subjective phenomenon and traditional tests, such as vibrametry and nerve conduction studies, have only measured function in large myelinated fibres. Recently, neurophysiological tests have been developed that enable clinical assessment of the peripheral and central nociceptive system.

Quantitative sensory testing (QST) measures detection thresholds (i.e. sensory responses) to thermal and electrical stimuli. The most sensitive of these is thermal threshold sensitivity (TTS) testing which involves the application of a thermode to the skin. When the thermode is heated or cooled, the patient indicates detection and pain thresholds for both warmth and cold; markers of C and Aδ fibre function respectively. Comparison with a non-painful control site enables the presence of sensory loss as well as allodynia to be determined.

Measuring the perception threshold to electrical currents is another method of assessing peripheral nerve function. Commercially available devices deliver a current at three different frequencies that are designed to stimulate C, Aδ, and Aβ fibres and comparisons are made with control sites and pooled normal data.

Tests of the autonomic system include the quantitative sudomotor axon reflex test (QSART) which measures the latency and volume of sweat from a given skin surface in response to activation of an axon reflex. This test demonstrates autonomic dysfunction but does not indicate that this is the underlying mechanism of neuropathic pain.

Microneurography and laser-evoked potentials (LEPs) are largely research techniques that objectively evaluate nociceptive pathway function. Microneurography assesses the response of primary afferent and sympathetic efferent neurons to electrical stimuli while LEPs test central responses to laser-evoked stimuli in the periphery. The laser technique has the advantage of being non-invasive.

Detailed laboratory tests are time-consuming and expensive and are not routinely used except in some clinical research studies. Minor changes in detection thresholds also occur in non-neuropathic pain conditions and so QST can only provide the clinician with a surrogate marker of neuropathic pain.

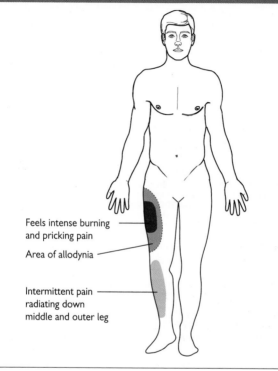

Fig 4.5 Example of a body-map illustrating sensory abnormalities associated with neuropathic pain caused by back injury

Feels intense burning and pricking pain

Area of allodynia

Intermittent pain radiating down middle and outer leg

4.5 **Verbal pain description**

4.5.1 **Role of verbal description**

Classical or textbook lists of symptoms and signs make for an easy diagnosis. The problem in practice is that most patients are not textbooks and the presentation of most disease, and pain in particular, takes some analysis.

As pain remains a subjective phenomenon and neuropathic pain is thought to result in unique sensations, it makes sense to use verbal description as a basis for distinguishing neuropathic pain from tissue injury pain. A number of studies have shown that patients with neuropathic pain select certain pain descriptors with more frequency than those with nociceptive pain. This led to the development of several scales to systematically assess this information.

Verbal pain descriptor scales can contribute important information to the assessment process alongside clinical history, examination, and investigation. These scales also provide standardized symptom assessments for patients in research studies that examine treatment effects or measure change in painful conditions over time.

4.5.2 Neuropathic pain scale (NPS)

This was the first scale to measure the intensity of 11 features that were thought to be reflective of neuropathic pain. These included generic features such as overall pain intensity, unpleasantness, and periodicity (intermittent, constant, flare-ups) as well as more specific features such as sharp, itchy, burning, and surface pain. The scale was not intended to distinguish neuropathic pain from nociceptive pain but has been widely used to measure changes in intensity of neuropathic pain symptoms. In particular, the NPS has shown sensitivity to treatment effects.

4.5.3 Leeds Assessment of Neuropathic Symptoms and Signs (LANSS) pain scale

The LANSS was the first tool that attempted to discriminate between neuropathic pain and nociceptive pain. In this regard, it has around 80% accuracy when compared to expert clinician assessment. The LANSS consists of five symptom items and two clinical examination items (allodynia and pinprick testing), and takes around five minutes to complete. The LANSS has been used extensively in the UK and internationally and has been validated in a number of independent studies examining cancer neuropathic pain, fibromyalgia, low back pain, and pain clinic populations. It has also shown sensitivity to treatment effects: for example, patients with intractable neuropathic pain (trigeminal neuralgia or post-stroke pain) showed reduction in LANSS score after successful treatment with transcranial magnetic stimulation, but not with placebo.

The LANSS has been further developed into a patient self-report tool, the S-LANSS score (see Appendix 2). This allows wider use and offers opportunities to conduct large-scale studies, including epidemiological research (see Chapter 3).

4.5.4 Other scales

In recent years, other scales similar to the NPS and LANSS have been published that attempt to improve upon their accuracy and utility. These include the Neuropathic Pain Questionnaire (NPQ) and the Douleur Neuropathique 4 (DN4) (see Appendix 2). Both of these have not been extensively validated in prospective studies and have not shown superior diagnostic accuracy or acceptability to the NPS and LANSS.

Alongside qualitative verbal description, generic information on pain intensity (such as visual analogue scores) and its impact on daily living (often called 'interference') also form part of the patient assessment. These aspects are not discussed in detail here.

4.6 **Can pain be more or less neuropathic?**

When assessing a patient with chronic pain, it is tempting to think that their underlying pain mechanism is either nociceptive or neuropathic, and current taxonomy encourages this view. However, experienced clinicians know that this is an oversimplification. In reality, patients present with a variety of clinical features, including anatomical and physiological abnormalities, which form a very mixed picture.

An emerging view is that pain, and chronic pain in particular, can be more or less neuropathic. In other words, the features of chronic pain experienced by any patient reflect the balance between underlying nociceptive and neuropathic mechanisms. From a clinical perspective, the diagnostic question is not 'is this pain neuropathic or nociceptive?' but 'what is the dominance of neuropathic mechanisms within this chronic pain state?' Although this view offers a more flexible clinical model and therefore opens up treatment opportunities, it requires further validation and testing.

Key references

Attal, N. and Bouhassira, D. (2004). Can pain be more or less neuropathic? *Pain*, **110**, 510–11.

Bennett, M. (2001). The LANSS pain scale: the Leeds Assessment of Neuropathic Symptoms and Signs. *Pain*, **92**, 147–57.

Bennett, M.I., Smith, B.H., Torrance, N., Lee, A.J. (2006). Can pain be more or less neuropathic? Comparison of symptom assessment tools with ratings of certainty by clinicians. *Pain*, 122 (3):289–294.

Bennett, M.I., Smith, B.H., Torrance, N., and Potter, J. (2005). The S-LANSS score for identifying pain of predominantly neuropathic origin: validation for use in clinic and postal research. *J. Pain*, **6**, 149–58.

Cruccu, G., Anand, P., Attal, N., Garcia-Larrea, L., Haanpaa, M., Jorum, E., et al. (2004). EFNS guidelines on neuropathic pain assessment. *Eur. J. Neurol.*, **11**, 153–62.

Galer, B.S. and Jensen, M.P. (1997). Development and preliminary validation of a pain measure specific to neuropathic pain: the Neuropathic Pain Scale. *Neurology*, **48**, 332–8.

Hansson, P. (2003). Difficulties in stratifying neuropathic pain by mechanisms. *Eur. J. Pain*, **7**, 353–7.

Jensen, T.S. and Baron, R. (2003). Translation of symptoms and signs into mechanisms in neuropathic pain. *Pain*, **102**, 1–8.

Chapter 5

Peripheral neuropathic pain

Tim Nash

Key points

- Damage to peripheral nerves, including cranial nerves and spinal nerve roots, can result in peripheral neuropathic pain.
- Speed of onset and associated symptoms and signs can point towards possible causes.
- Common conditions include diabetic neuropathy, post-herpetic neuralgia, and post-surgical neuropathies including phantom limb pain.
- Less common conditions result from Guillain-Barré syndrome, deficiency states, and toxic neuropathies.
- Treatment is based on co-analgesics with or without opioids. Some conditions, such as trigeminal neuralgia and other compression problems, can respond well to decompression surgery.

5.1 Introduction

5.1.1 Role of peripheral nociceptive system

It is a commonly held belief that the pain system has an important role in alerting the individual to the threat of tissue damage. Pain is not normally felt until after the injury has occurred, and frequently not until some time after the injury. It is therefore questionable as to whether pain has any value. Neuropathic pain particularly has no value, the pain developing and persisting as a result of damage to or dysfunction of the nervous system, persisting after all possible healing has occurred.

5.1.2 Sites of peripheral damage

Peripheral neuropathic pain can result from any damage to or dysfunction of the peripheral nervous system, which includes the cranial nerves (except the optic nerve), spinal nerve roots, dorsal root ganglia, peripheral nerve trunks, and nerve terminals. Disruption of the somatosensory system results in loss of sensation and analgesia in the affected area. This can affect motor, sensory, autonomic, or mixed nerve fibres, and may lead to aberrant somatosensory processing, with the paradox of pain in the hypo-aesthetic area (see Chapter 2).

5.1.3 Painless neuropathies

Neuropathies such as leprosy, congenital insensitivity to pain (Hereditary Sensory and Autonomic Neuropathy), and Tangier disease (familial high protein density lipoprotein deficiency), are painless because of the predominant loss of pain sensation. A common misconception is that it is this absence of pain sensation that often leads to severe mutilation. Sternbach pointed out in 1963 that where other sensory cues persisted in patients with congenital insensitivity to pain, they were able to avoid such harm.

5.2 Clinical manifestations

5.2.1 Symptoms and history

Despite the varied conditions, site, and type of nerve damage, the clinical picture in peripheral neuropathic pain is generally very similar (see also Chapter 4).

The pain may include the following features:

- it may be spontaneous, and can be paroxysmal, lasting for seconds up to minutes, several times a day to a few times every week
- paroxysmal pain may be shooting, intense, or sharp
- it may be constantly burning, aching, or sore
- typically there is also evoked pain, mostly caused by lightly touching the skin or by exposure to wind (allodynia)
- frequently dysaesthesia (numbness, pins and needles) is present.

The pain may vary spontaneously, but typically intensifies with activity and exposure to cold. There may be increased sympathetic activity.

Common features of peripheral neuropathic pain include a history of:

- possible neurological injury (surgery or trauma)
- spontaneous or paroxysmal pain
- pain in distribution of a nerve (neuralgia)
- pain persisting after tissue healing
- descriptors such as burning, electrical, shooting, stabbing
- poor response to opioids, with steadily increasing opioid requirement.

The speed of onset of the neuropathy can give a guide as to its aetiology (Table 5.1).

Table 5.1 Likely causes of neuropathy according to speed of onset

Acute onset	Inflammatory
	Immunological
	Toxic
	Vascular
Subacute onset over weeks or months	Toxic
	Nutritional
	Systemic disease
Chronic onset over many years	Hereditary
	Metabolic disease

5.2.2 Clinical examination of peripheral nerves

This should assess the presence of:

- allodynia (pain elicited by a stimulus that does not normally provoke pain)
- hyperpathia (abnormally painful reaction to a stimulus, especially a repeated stimulus, often explosive, radiating, and with after-sensations)
- hypoaesthesia (decreased sensitivity to stimulation)
- hyperaesthesia (increased sensitivity to stimulation)
- hypoalgesia (diminished pain in response to a normally painful stimulus)
- hyperalgesia (increased pain in response to a normally painful stimulus)
- paraesthesia (unpleasant abnormal sensation, spontaneous or provoked)
- neurological deficit (e.g. nerve root avulsion)
- autonomic/vasomotor dysfunction (e.g. unilateral skin temperature changes)
- Tinel's sign (tapping damaged peripheral nerves, causes shocks radiating in nerve distribution).

Establishing a diagnosis may enable treatment of the cause and consequent improvement in the pain. Diagnostic tests for peripheral neuropathic pain are summarized in Table 5.2.

Table 5.2 Tests used to aid diagnosis of peripheral neuropathies		
Diagnostic test	Investigates	Establishes
Nerve conduction and Electromyography	Large-fibre function only	Nerve disorder: <ul><li>generalized polyneuropathy</li><li>multifocal neuropathy</li><li>mononeuropathy</li><li>distinguishes between primary demyelinating neuropathy and axonal neuropathy</li></ul>
Quantitative sensory testing	Nerve fibre function: <ul><li>small myelinated</li><li>small unmyelinated</li><li>large myelinated</li></ul>	Can particularly show pure small-fibre neuropathy
Blood tests	Blood sugar Vitamin assays Lead and other assays Immunoglobulins and anti-neural antibody	Metabolic disease Nutritional deficiency Toxicity states Immune-mediated neuropathies
Genetic screening		Inherited neuropathies
Cerebrospinal fluid assessment	Protein Cellular response	Radicular or meningeal involvement
Nerve and muscle biopsy	Nerve/muscle pathology	Mononeuritis multiplex: <ul><li>vasculitis</li><li>amyloidosis</li><li>leprosy</li><li>subacute or chronic distal symmetric polyneuropathies</li></ul> Genetically determined paediatric disorders

Examination findings may suggest that the peripheral neuropathy is symmetrical or asymmetrical and this can point towards possible causes (Tables 5.3 and 5.4).

Table 5.3 Pathological causes of symmetrical painful neuropathies and neuropathic pain

Metabolic	Diabetes mellitus
	Hypoglycaemic (insulinoma)
	Hypothyroidism
Nutritional/deficiency	Pellagra (niacin deficiency)
	Beriberi (thiamine deficiency)
	Multiple nutritional deficiencies
Toxic	Drugs:
	• alcohol
	• antiretroviral drugs
	• cytotoxic
	• isoniazid, hydralazine, etc.
	Metals:
	• thallium
	• arsenic
	• mercury
Immune mediated	Acute/chronic inflammatory demyelinating
	Associated with:
	• paraproteinaemia
	• cryoglobinaemia
	• acquired amyloidosis
	Paraneoplastic
Hereditary	Hereditary sensory and autonomic neuropathy (type 1)
	Fabry's disease
Idiopathic	

Table 5.4 Pathological causes of asymmetrical painful neuropathies and neuropathic pain

Mononeuritis/mononeuritis multiplex	Diabetic:
	• cranial neuropathy
	• trunk/limb mononeuropathy
	• amyotrophy
	Vasculitic:
	• systemic of vasa nervorum:
	  • polyarteritis nodosa
	  • churg-Strauss syndrome
	  • rheumatoid arthritis
	  • lupus erythematosus
	  • systemic sclerosis
	  • wegener's granulomatosis
	• isolated angiitis of peripheral nerves
	Infectious/para-infectious:
	• HIV related
	• borreliosis
	• herpes zoster

Physical injury	Nerve entrapment: • carpal tunnel and other nerve compression • root compression (intervertebral disk herniation) • neuroma (post-traumatic, post-surgical, post-amputation Radiation induced Post-traumatic plexus neuropathy Tumour infiltration Phantom limb pain
Idiopathic neuritis	Brachial neuritis Lumbosacral neuritis
Cranial neuralgias	Trigeminal neuralgia Glossopharyngeal neuralgia

5.3 **Well-recognized causes of peripheral neuropathic pain**

5.3.1 **Diabetic neuropathy**

This is the most common cause of neuropathy in the Western world, affecting about 50% of diabetic patients over time. It is usually seen in diabetics over 50 years old, and is related directly to the toxic effects of hyperglycaemia. The effects of glucose metabolism may also be responsible.

The most common form of neuropathy in diabetes mellitus is a distal symmetrical polyneuropathy, which is predominantly sensory. The main complaint is persisting distressing numbness and tingling, worse at night, often confined to the feet and lower legs. A deep aching may develop, with lancinating pain and burning. There is initial distal reduction in light touch, pain, and vibration sensation, but as the neuropathy progresses this extends more proximally and may involve the hands and trunk. Ankle jerks are reduced and mild weakness may occur. Painless foot ulceration together with autonomic neuropathy develops in severe cases with universal severe dysfunction of all nerve fibre populations due to demyelination with or without axonal degeneration. The upper limbs may also be involved.

Rarely, an acute painful diabetic neuropathy can present with profound weight loss and burning pain that is worse at night. This can follow an episode of ketosis or establishment of tight glycaemic control. There is little sensory or motor loss, but there is hyperalgesia and contact with clothing and bedding is unpleasant. Symptoms tend to improve with weight gain and adequate diabetic control. Occasionally, paraesthesiae and pain follow the institution of insulin therapy, but this tends to improve slowly with glycaemic control.

Painful asymmetric neuropathy, probably due to a vasculitis affecting small epineural vessels, is sometimes seen in older patients with mild or undetected diabetes. Pain often starts in the back or hip and spreads down the leg on one side. There is usually weakness and wasting of the pelvic girdle and thigh muscles. Recovery is normal, but may be incomplete. Acute diabetic mononeuropathy may result from infarction of a nerve.

Diabetic thoracolumbar radiculopathy due to a lesion proximal in the nerve root occurs in older patients with long-standing diabetes and may be associated with weight loss. It presents with girdle pain around the trunk, either unilateral or bilateral, and there may be abdominal wall weakness, cutaneous hyperaesthesia, or superficial sensory loss over the affected area. EMG changes can be detected in paraspinal and abdominal wall muscles. Recovery may be protracted, but ultimate prognosis is good.

5.3.2 **Post-herpetic neuralgia**

Shingles (herpes zoster infection) is frequently painful. Pain may persist in the affected area for more than 12 weeks following the healing of the herpetic skin lesions, especially in the elderly (50% of patients over 50 years old), to become post-herpetic neuralgia. It can be severe and debilitating, and may abate after months or continue for years.

Both peripheral and central mechanisms are involved. Minimal sensory loss characteristically produces abnormal sensitization of unmyelinated cutaneous nociceptors. Small-fibre deafferentation may profoundly impair pain and temperature sensation, giving allodynia to a moving stimulus (dynamic allodynia), almost certainly due to the formation of new connections between non-nociceptive large-diameter primary afferents and central pain transmission neurons. Deafferentation with loss of both large- and small-diameter fibres will give increased spontaneous activity in deafferented central neurons with or without reorganization of central connections, and severe spontaneous pain with hyperalgesia or allodynia. Each of these changes may be present to different degrees in any patient.

5.3.3 **Trigeminal neuralgia**

Trigeminal neuralgia is a sudden, usually unilateral, severe, brief, stabbing, recurrent pain in the distribution of one or more branches of the fifth cranial nerve. Eighty per cent (80%) of cases are idiopathic, and 66% of these have vascular pressure at the root entry zone. Other causes include demyelinating plaques in multiple sclerosis, angioma, brainstem infarcts, and tumours such as acoustic neuromas.

5.3.4 **Post-surgical neuropathic pain**

Post-surgical neuropathic pain can result from surgical section with deafferentation, compression, stretching, ischaemia, and infection of the nerve. It has been estimated that 10% of all surgery produces post-surgical neuropathic pain, including painful scars. During the process of regeneration of nerves, the axonal sprouts generate neural activity, which is most marked when neuromata develop. The consequent barrage of activity into the spinal cord leads to central sensitization.

5.3.5 **Phantom limb pain**

From very early childhood virtually everyone who has an amputation experiences sensations apparently arising from the amputated limb or organ. As time passes the phantom limb becomes less vivid, and the limb appears to telescope into the amputation stump, although most feel the phantom for the rest of their lives. Phantom limb pain is common, 80% of amputees having troublesome pain for at least one week every year, and many for considerably more of the year. The pain is frequently exacerbated by irritation in the stump, exhaustion, back pain, stress, or external factors such as changes in humidity.

5.3.6 Post-traumatic neuropathic pain

Traumatic lesions, such as brachial plexus avulsion from the spinal cord, frequently produce an intractable, persistent, severe, disabling pain that is a constant crushing and intermittent shooting pain.

5.3.7 Human immunodeficiency virus (HIV)

Various types of peripheral neuropathy may complicate HIV infection, producing pain in 30% of patients with HIV, the most common being a distal symmetrical polyneuropathy as a direct result of the infection. HIV-1 is highly neurotrophic and is present in the central nervous system in the earliest stages of infection, well before significant immunosuppression. Neuropathy can occur from the antiretroviral drugs, vitamin B_{12} deficiency associated with HIV, and concurrent alcoholism. Painful mononeuropathy multiplex related to focal vasculitis, or subacute cauda equina syndrome, or radiculopathy due to cytomegalovirus infection also occurs. Inflammatory demyelinating neuropathies may produce Guillain-Barré syndrome. Clearly, antiretroviral treatment may be helpful.

5.3.8 Nerve compression and entrapment neuropathies

A nerve may be mechanically constricted in a fibro-osseous tunnel or deformed by a fibrous band. Symptoms come on gradually (sensory more than motor, except in the elderly) and fluctuate with activity and rest. Systemic conditions should always be excluded that can make nerves prone to compression, such as diabetes, hypothyroidism, pregnancy, and amyloid, and hereditary liability to pressure palsies. Common sites are shown in Box 5.1.

Box 5.1 Common sites for entrapment neuropathies

- Median nerve compression at wrist
- Ulnar nerve in cubital canal at the elbow or in Guyon's canal at the wrist
- Suprascapular nerve at spinoglenoid notch
- Posterior interosseous nerve in the radial tunnel
- Lateral femoral cutaneous nerve of the thigh (meralgia paraesthetica) at the inguinal ligament
- Obturator nerve in the obturator canal
- Posterior tibial nerve in the tarsal tunnel
- Interdigital plantar nerve (Morton's metatarsalgia) in the plantar fascia between the heads of the third and fourth metatarsals

5.3.9 Complex regional pain syndrome

Complex regional pain syndrome (CRPS) is associated with trauma, either mild with no nerve injury (type 1), or more major with nerve injury (type 2). Allodynia, hyperpathia, and autonomic signs are present. Autonomic changes are significant (see Chapter 7).

5.3.10 Cancer

Neuropathic pain can occur in cancer, frequently due to tumour invasion, but also because of radiation fibrosis, radiation myelopathy, chemotherapy, or surgery (especially after mastectomy or thoracotomy). If standard analgesic, adjunctive, and neuropathic drug therapy is inadequate, then interventions can be useful, such as spinal drug delivery systems, or neurodestructive techniques such as intrathecal neurolysis or percutaneous cordotomy. Paraneoplastic neuropathies occur as remote effects of carcinoma and can precede detection of malignancy by months or years (see Chapter 8).

5.4 Less well-recognized causes

5.4.1 Guillain-Barré syndrome

Acute inflammatory neuropathies can affect cranial, respiratory, and upper limbs early in the course of the disease, generally as an autoimmune response. Guillain-Barré syndrome, a demyelinating polyneuropathy, may have an autoimmune base following an infection, and affects peripheral nerves predominantly, concentrating on the region where the anterior and posterior spinal roots fuse. It is always bilateral but not always symmetrical, and produces motor paralysis or weakness and sensory deficit. Generally recovery occurs. Pain, paraesthesiae, and dysaesthesiae commonly occur, although motor abnormalities predominate.

5.4.2 Other autoimmune neuropathies

Polyarteritis nodosa, Churg-Strauss syndrome, rheumatoid arthritis, lupus erythematosus, systemic sclerosis, and Wegener's granulomatosis can produce a vasculitic neuropathy, usually a mononeuritis multiplex. Cryoglobulinaemia may produce a mononeuritis multiplex or symmetrical polyneuropathy with painful dysaesthesiae. Primary amyloidosis presents with painful dysaesthesiae and numbness, with disturbance of small-fibre activity in pain, temperature, and autonomic small-fibres.

Neuralgic amyotrophy may develop suddenly in an otherwise healthy individual or follow an infection, surgical procedure, childbirth, or an injection of vaccine or antibiotic to produce a brachial neuralgia. It usually begins with a severe pain around the shoulder on one side, followed rapidly by profound weakness and atrophy, usually of the C5 and C6 myotomes. Movement of the involved muscles exacerbates the pain. Pain usually settles in a few days or weeks, and recovery is normally good.

5.4.3 Hypothyroid neuropathy

There is a high incidence of carpal tunnel syndrome in hypothyroidism, but a sensorimotor polyneuropathy can also occur with painful dysaesthesiae and lancinating pains in the hands and feet, and glove and stocking sensory loss, with occasional distal weakness and wasting. It improves with thyroxine replacement therapy.

5.4.4 Deficiency states

Neuropathy due to nutritional deficiency is uncommon in the developed world, and is usually seen in association with alcoholism, malabsorption, gastrointestinal surgery to produce weight loss in obesity, and prolonged stay in intensive care units. The common deficiency states are vitamins B_1 (thiamine), B_6 (pyridoxine) (associated with antituberculous treatment with isoniazid, and antihypertensive treatment with hydralazine), and niacin. Extremely high doses of pyridoxine may also cause a neuropathy. Alcoholic neuropathy is considered to be due to vitamin B_1 deficiency, and symptoms are non-specific.

5.4.5 Toxic neuropathies

Arsenic ingestion will produce a systemic illness (gastrointestinal symptoms, anaemia, jaundice, hyperkeratosis of palms and soles, and later white transverse banding of nails), with associated neuropathy and aching or burning pain, tingling, or numbness in the fingers and toes spreading proximally.

Thallium ingestion will produce a rapidly progressing painful sensory neuropathy, whereas mercury will affect the central nervous system (visual field defects, ataxia, mental impairment), but a polyneuropathy can develop early with distal paraesthesiae that may involve the tongue.

Peripheral neuropathy is the significant dose-limiting side-effect of many cytotoxic and antiretroviral drugs. Ten per cent (10%) of patients on zalcitabine or stavudine have to discontinue therapy with the development of neuropathy.

5.4.6 Hereditary neuropathies

Hereditary sensory and autonomic neuropathy (HSAN) type 1, an autosomal dominant inherited condition, can produce spontaneous burning, aching, or lancinating pain. Fabry's disease may also present with burning sensations in the hands and lower legs, with tender legs in young boys or men, and pain so severe that walking is limited.

5.5 **Treatment options**

5.5.1 **Analgesics**

Frequently, neuropathic pain responds poorly to standard analgesics. Tricyclic antidepressants have useful efficacy, but their side-effects are problematic. Anti-epileptic drugs have similar efficacy and can be used with tricyclics or in combination with different anti-epileptics (see Chapter 9). Capsaicin cream is useful for allodynia. Opioids can be useful, especially in severe pain, and both tramadol and oxycodone have been shown to be useful in diabetic neuropathy (see Chapter 12).

5.5.2 **Non-drug options**

Neuromodulation using TENS, acupuncture, or spinal cord stimulation can also be helpful (see Chapters 13 and 14). TENS electrodes need to be applied over accessible functioning nerves proximal to the lesion, or over the painful area (which is usually too large to be practical) that has normal sensation. Acupuncture is not practical in the long term.

Trigeminal neuralgia, or other nerve compression problems, can respond well to decompression surgery, and trigeminal neuralgia can also be helped by per-foraminal ovale neurodestructive procedures. Neuropathic cancer pain can also respond to interventions such as spinal drug delivery systems or, if unilateral, percutaneous cordotomy can be invaluable.

Key references

Fields, H.L., Rowbotham, M., and Baron, R. (1998). Postherpetic neuralgia: irritable nociceptors and deafferentation. *Neurobiol. Disease*, **5**, 209–27.

Grady, K.M., Severn, A.M., and Eldridge, P.R. (2002). *Key topics in chronic pain* (2nd edn). Taylor & Francis, Abingdon.

Jensen, T.S. and Gottrup, H. (2003). Assessment of neuropathic pain. In: T.S. Jensen, P.R. Wilson, and A.S.C. Rice (ed.) *Clinical pain management: chronic pain,* pp. 113–24. Arnold, London.

Shembalkar, P. and Anand, P. (2003). Peripheral neuropathies. In: T.S. Jensen, P.R. Wilson, and A.S.C. Rice (ed.) *Clinical pain management: chronic pain,* pp. 355–66. Arnold, London.

Sternbach, R.A. (1963). Congenital insensitivity to pain: a critique. *Psychol Bull* 1963; 60: 252–64.

Chapter 6

Central neuropathic pain

David Bowsher

Key points

- Central neuropathic pain can arise following damage to spinothalamocortical pathways in the spinal cord and brain.
- Stroke, multiple sclerosis, and spinal cord injury (trauma or disease) are the predominant causes.
- Central neuropathic pain is wrongly considered a rarity; several tens of thousands of cases exist in the UK and it can develop up to two years after stroke.
- Tactile and cold allodynia are common.
- Central neuropathic pain seems to be less responsive to co-analgesics and opioids than peripheral neuropathic pain, though substantial pain relief can be achieved in a proportion.

6.1 Background

Most health professionals, on seeing the phrase 'central neuropathic pain', think immediately of central post-stroke pain (CPSP), or as it erroneously used to be called, thalamic syndrome. In fact, central neuropathic pain (CNP) occurs after a number of other central nervous system insults. High on the list are spinal cord injury (SCI) and syringomyelia, as well as some other supraspinal conditions such as Wallenberg's syndrome and multiple sclerosis. Central neuropathic pain has been defined as pain arising from damage to the ascending spinothalamocortical pathways, their relays, or end-stations in the spinal cord or brain. This seems to the present author to be the best and most comprehensive definition of CNP. Furthermore, CNP shares with peripheral neuropathic pains the useful clinical definition of 'pain in an area of altered sensation'.

6.2 **Epidemiology of central neuropathic pain**

6.2.1 **Stroke and spinal cord injury**

Central post-stroke pain is the form of CNP with which most pain practitioners are most frequently concerned. CPSP was originally called 'thalamic syndrome' because the first cases described almost 100 years ago had lesions in the thalamus, or more precisely, in the posterolateroventral thalamic nucleus, and so the name 'thalamic syndrome' became sanctified. Leaving aside the large number of cerebral stroke lesions outside the thalamus which are now known to cause CPSP, it has more recently been shown that only 25% of patients with classical (posterolateroventral thalamic) lesions develop CPSP (Fig. 6.1).

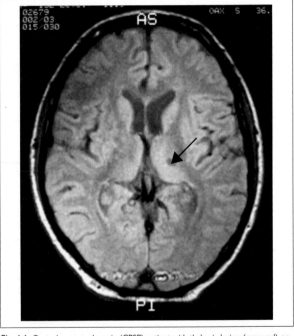

Fig. 6.1 Central post-stroke pain (CPSP) patient with thalamic lesion (arrowed) on left. *Clinical features*: right-sided burning pain, raised tactile (von Frey), warm, cool, and hot pain thresholds; mechanical pain threshold (skin-fold pinch) not raised. No allodynia.

There are about 100,000 strokes per year in the UK and one-third of these are fatal. Of the rest, the incidence of CPSP is about 8–10,000 cases per year. Since most cases of CPSP are in patients who do not have very severe motor deficits, the patients tend to have quite a good survival rate, so that the prevalence of CPSP in the UK is probably of the order of 50,000. In the USA, these figures may be multiplied by five, so that there may be a quarter of a million CPSP sufferers.

CNP probably affects two-thirds of patients with SCI. The prevalence of SCI is not accurately recorded, but there are of course a large number of cases, caused not only by extreme sports but in the main by traffic accidents. Similarly, around 30% of patients with multiple sclerosis develop CNP, though the exact prevalence is hard to determine.

6.2.2 **CNP in the population**

Given the very large numbers of patients with CNP (tens of thousands of cases in the UK and hundreds of thousands in North America), it remains a matter of mystery as to why CNP is regarded as a rarity by health professionals. The fact that it has multiple causes may contribute to this notion, and possibly interfere intellectually with its treatment as an entity.

It has already been stated that one-third of patients with spinal cord injuries do not have CNP. While figures for other forms of CNP are not so well established, the failure to develop neuropathic pain in a large number of subjects with many forms of damage to the peripheral or central nervous system is perhaps what should really be occupying our attention when seeking a pathophysiological explanation for the condition.

6.3 **Features of central neuropathic pain**

6.3.1 **Pain**

This may be permanent or intermittent, constant or fluctuating in intensity. Descriptions vary according to the individual patient, and of course to the language and culture group to which the patient belongs. Textbooks and teachers are very fond of saying that the pain is characteristically 'burning', but this is because other pains are not so described – not more than 50% of CNP patients use the word 'burning'. The pain may be aching or throbbing, stabbing or lancinating, like many non-neuropathic pains. The nearest most healthy people get to it is sunburn, which is a *temporary* neuropathic pain due to reversible nerve damage, or to holding a snowball in the hand for too long – 'ice-burn'.

Nearly half of stroke patients who have CNP feel pain on regaining consciousness, and 60% develop the pain within three months.

However, the rest take up to two years to develop pain. This means that a large proportion of CNP patients will have been discharged from specialized care by the time they develop CNP. Family practitioners and nurses should therefore be on the lookout for late-developing CNP in stroke patients. CNP onset following SCI is also not immediate in many cases.

6.3.2 Altered sensation

The painful area always occurs *within* (i.e. is smaller than) an area of altered superficial skin sensation. The sensations most frequently changed (i.e. with raised thresholds) are innocuous and noxious temperature sensations, sharpness, and mechanical pain. That is, the sensations subserved by smaller peripheral nerve fibres are the most affected. Pain intensity seems to correlate in particular with the degree of innocuous temperature deficit. Tactile and vibratory sensations are less frequently affected.

Testing for innocuous changes

Raised thresholds for innocuous temperature means inability to appreciate warmth in something slightly warmer than the patient's skin, such as the examiner's finger; or slightly cooler, such as a metal spoon or tuning fork. It does not mean near-boiling or iced water in a test-tube. Similarly, sharpness does not mean shoving a pin or needle deep into the tissues and twisting it – that's painful! Sharpness is tested by seeing whether the patient, with eyes closed, can tell the difference between the head and the point of a pin gently applied to the skin surface.

Testing for mechanical and thermal pain

Mechanical pain can be tested by grasping and squeezing a skin fold between finger and thumb, and heat pain with a test-tube containing water (or any other object) at 50–60°. It is very important to specify whether mechanical or thermal pain is affected; there is no such thing as 'pain' (unspecified), nor of course is there such a thing as 'painful stimulation'. *Noxious* (potentially tissue-damaging) stimulation, either mechanical or thermal, *would* result in a sensation of pain in a normal intact person, but not in the unconscious person or a patient with lost sensation in the stimulated area.

Heat and mechanical pains are in different categories from the periphery onwards. This is illustrated in the periphery by the fact that application of capsaicin abolishes response to painful or noxious heat, but not to painful or noxious mechanical stimulation. The differentiation is maintained within the central nervous system, as shown by the fact that some central lesions interfere with appreciation of stimuli of one noxious type but not the other (Fig. 6.2).

Since Nature conveniently provides a control in all cases, responses to sensory tests should be compared between the affected area and the mirror-image unaffected area on the other side.

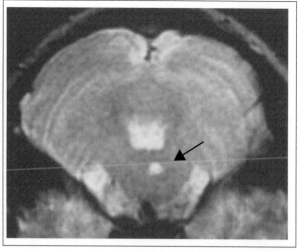

Fig. 6.2 Pontine lesion. Lesion in pons (arrowed), just below fourth ventricle, above which is the cerebellum. *Clinical features*: throbbing pain in left side, tactile (von Frey) threshold unaffected; mechanical pain threshold (skin-fold pinch) raised; warm and cool thresholds minimally (perhaps non-significantly) raised; hot pain threshold significantly raised. No allodynia.

6.3.3 **Allodynia**

This is defined as pain experienced on stimulation by a non-noxious stimulus. Allodynia usually occurs within the painful area, and is encountered in about 70% of patients with CPSP. The commonest form is tactile allodynia, which is elicited by light brushing and occurs in 50% of cases. Less common are cold allodynia, elicited by non-noxious cold stimulation, and movement allodynia, elicited by active or passive stretching of muscles or tendons. Unlike the sensations whose thresholds are most frequently raised, the sensations most frequently causing allodynia are those subserved by large peripheral nerve fibres, thus demonstrating the important interactions between afferent fibres of different sizes at the first or subsequent synapses within the central nervous system. More than one form of allodynia may occur in the same patient.

Just occasionally, allodynia within the painful area can be elicited by appropriate stimulation at some distant body site, but always on the same side as the CNP pain. Patients usually volunteer this recondite information (e.g. 'My chest hurts every time I brush the side of my calf') because it's so unusual, unexpected, and inexplicable.

6.3.4 **Autonomic component**

When large body areas are involved, such as a whole limb in CPSP, the affected area may feel cold, both subjectively and objectively. This is evidence of an autonomic component to CNP. The coldness (vasoconstriction) can be got rid of by prescribing a calcium-channel blocker, but as this doesn't relieve the pain, it's not worth doing unless the cold sensation in itself really disturbs the patient.

6.3.5 **Site of the lesion**

The intellectual challenge of locating the site of the lesion has been removed by the universality of imaging. But for those who wish to use imaging as confirmation of their diagnosis, the following may be borne in mind with regard to CNP:

- *history* – ?stroke; ?injury; ?sudden or gradual onset
- *distribution of pain and sensory change* – there should be no difficulty in distinguishing infra- from supraspinal causes of CNP. In supraspinal CNP, lesions above the decussation of the medial lemniscus in the upper medulla oblongata give rise to both pain and sensory loss on the contralateral side. Low medullary lesions, however, cause loss of soft touch sensation in the ipsilateral face (trigeminal nerve palsy) but pain and temperature loss in the contralateral limb(s): Wallenberg's syndrome.

In cases where all symptoms occur on the side opposite the lesion, if the greatest pain and/or deficit occurs in the extremities, the lesion is most probably in the thalamus or cortex; but if the greatest pain or deficit is not in the extremities, the lesion is probably infrathalamic. If the most severe pain is in the face, the lesion is probably infratentorial.

6.4 **Possible mechanisms of CNP**

It had earlier been suggested that one mechanism of CNP might lie in the level of particular, but unknown, transmitters and/or receptors in the central nervous system. Thus if certain transmitters or receptors are depleted as a result of insult to the central nervous system, CNP might ensue. A similar suggestion with regard to pain following SCI has also been made. If the depletion is sudden and massive, immediate pain occurs; if gradual, pain develops gradually. If levels of transmitters or receptors are up-regulated by treatment or by Nature, recovery takes place. This hypothesis is supported by a number of investigations involving specific receptors, such as NK_1 serotonin receptors, spinal $5HT_3$ receptors, or transmitters such as ubiquitin C-terminal hydrolase. However, it should be noted that the above hypothesis does not explain why CNP is sometimes relieved by the occurrence of a further stroke, resulting in yet more damage to the brain.

6.5 **Treatment**

6.5.1 **Co-analgesics**

Up to about the 1970s, CNP was mainly treated by the administration of larger and larger doses of stronger and stronger analgesics, including morphine and heroin. The unfortunate result of this was the existence of a large number of agonized junkies. In the 1960s, it was found that trigeminal neuralgia (now known not to be a typical form of neuropathic pain) could be relieved by carbamazepine and subsequently other antiepileptics. Thus began the treatment of CNP with a mixture of analgesics and anti-epileptics, resulting in overweight, cognitively challenged patients.

Alongside this, however, it had been found that tricyclic antidepressants of the amitriptyline group, which had noradrenergic as well as serotonergic properties, were effective in the treatment of neuropathic pain of peripheral origin, particularly post-herpetic neuralgia. This finding was applied with some success to the treatment of CPSP, in which it was found, as in post-herpetic neuralgia, that the sooner after pain onset such treatment was initiated, the greater the possibility of success. If treatment was commenced within six months of pain onset, almost 90% were relieved; and within 12 months, two-thirds; subsequent to this, the proportion fell to less than half.

Ami- and nortriptyline, which often have undesirable side-effects, are noradrenergic and serotonergic. Pure serotonergic antidepressants, such as fluoxetine, although having many fewer adverse effects, are unfortunately virtually useless in the treatment of CNP.

However, the idea of effective anti-epileptic treatment, despite the failure of carbamazepine, continued to haunt many physicians; and modern anti-epileptics such as gabapentin and pregabalin, together with lamotrigine, have been found to produce pain relief in a proportion of cases.

6.5.2 **Other approaches**

Modern pharmacotherapy has re-evaluated opioid treatment in a much more careful way. A number of judiciously applied opioids, such as oxycodone, or a mixture of dextromethorphan and morphine, have been successfully deployed in a proportion of cases. Membrane-stabilizing drugs, such as mexiletine, have been shown to be useful in the treatment of cases not responding to tricyclics.

In our series of over 100 cases of CPSP treated by non-opioid pharmacotherapy, about half achieved total or substantial relief of their pain. In intractable cases (of which, sadly, there are far too many), a number of interventional techniques have been, and are being, tried. For instance, electrical stimulation of the spinal cord or brain has met with a certain degree of success.

It is to be hoped that a better understanding of the molecular mechanisms of CNP will lead to more rational and effective treatment.

Key references

Beric, A., Dimitrijevic, M.R., Lindblom, U. (1988). Central dysesthesia syndrome in spinal cord injury patients. *Pain*, **34**, 109–116.

Bogousslavsky, J., Regli, F., Uske, A. (1988). Thalamic infarcts: clinical syndromes, etiology, and prognosis. *Neurology*, **38**, 837–848.

Boivie, J. (2006). Central Pain. In: McMahon, S.B., and Koltzenburg, M. (ed.) *Wall & Melzack's Textbook of Pain*, 5th edn., **67**, 1057–1074. Elsevier Churchill Livingstone.

Bowsher, D. (1996). *Central Pain: Clinical and Physiological Characteristics. J. Neurol. Neurosurg. Psychiat.*, **61**, 62–69.

Bowsher, D., Leijon, G., and Thuomas, K-A. (1988). Central Post-Stroke Pain: Correlation of Magnetic Resonance Imaging with Clinical Pain Characteristics and Sensory Abnormalities. *Neurology*, **51**, 1352–1358.

Bowsher, D. (2005). Allodynia in relation to lesion site in central post-stroke pain. *J. Pain*, **6**, 736–40.

Cassinari, V., Pagni, C.A. (1969). *Central Pain: A Neurosurgical Survey.* Harvard University Press, Cambridge, MA.

Dejerine, J., Roussy, J. (1906). Le syndrome thalamique. *Rev Neurol*, **14**, 521–532.

Chapter 7

Complex regional pain syndrome

Dudley Bush

Key points

- Complex regional pain syndrome is the current name for previously called reflex sympathetic dystrophy (now CRPS type I) and causalgia (now CRPS type II).
- It occurs in distal limbs following trauma or surgery, is not related to intensity of initial insult, and is idiopathic in 10% of cases. There are around 10,000 cases in the UK and it is four times more common in females.
- Mechanisms underlying CRPS are complex but may involve neurogenic inflammation.
- Weakness and autonomic changes commonly accompany pain.
- Treatment is based on relief of pain (with co-analgesics, opioids, and neuromodulation) combined with restoration of function, so early referral and treatment is essential to prevent irreversible trophic changes and contractures.

7.1 Background

7.1.1 Clinical definitions

Complex regional pain syndrome (CRPS) is the current name for an uncommon condition in which severe spontaneous or evoked pain persists disproportionate to an initiating event. CRPS usually occurs in the distal limb following trauma or surgery, but can occur spontaneously in any area and is not related to the severity of the initiating noxious insult. There are usually accompanying features of altered sensation, swelling, vasomotor instability, motor abnormality, and osteoporosis. Originally described in relation to traumatic nerve injury by Weir Mitchell during the American Civil War, and later by Sudeck in 1900 after wrist fracture, the condition has been recognized for many years but has only recently been systematically

> ### Box 7.1 Clinical definition of complex regional pain syndrome
>
> - Presence of an initiating noxious event or cause of immobilization
>   - type I – without obvious nerve injury
>   - type II – with obvious nerve injury
> - Continuing pain, allodynia, or hyperalgesia disproportionate to the initiating event and not limited to a single nerve territory
> - Evidence at some time of oedema, changes in skin blood flow, or abnormal sudomotor activity or motor symptoms
> - Other diagnoses are excluded, for example missed fracture, connective tissue disease

classified and studied. Previous names include reflex sympathetic dystrophy (RSD), sympathetically maintained pain, algodystrophy, Sudeck's atrophy, and causalgia.

The clinical definition of CRPS was produced in 1994 by the International Association for the Study of Pain (IASP) in an attempt to improve recognition and diagnosis of the condition (Box 7.1). It was hoped that the previous overemphasis upon involvement of the sympathetic nervous system in diagnosis would be avoided and that the confusion in nomenclature would be reduced. Type II CRPS is similar to type I except that initiating trauma must involve nerve injury.

7.1.2 Epidemiology

In a US population, the incidence of CRPS has been found to be approximately five per 100,000 years at risk, with a prevalence of 21 per 100,000, and a female:male ratio of 4:1. Half of all cases follow trauma, more commonly of the upper limb, with rates of 7% to 37% following wrist fracture. Limb surgery is a common cause; estimates of incidence are 2–4% after arthroscopic knee surgery, 2–5% after carpal tunnel surgery, 13% after ankle surgery, and 1–13% after total knee arthroplasty. CRPS may occur in other locations or follow other initiating events, including myocardial infarction and stroke, and in 10% of cases no precipitating event can be identified.

7.2 Clinical features

7.2.1 Sensory disturbance

Pain and hyperalgesia (increased response to a nociceptive stimulus) are the main features of CRPS, with the majority of patients reporting pain at rest. Common pain descriptors are burning, aching, and shooting. Allodynia (pain upon light touch) is a common feature in CRPS and hypo-aesthesia (decreased sensitivity) is common.

Mechanical allodynia is reported by most CRPS patients and manifests as pain upon movement. The sensory changes often do not occur in a neuroanatomical distribution and can become widespread.

7.2.2 Motor disturbance

Weakness is very common in CRPS, initially because of pain-dependent guarding, but later tremor, myoclonus, and focal dystonia are seen. Many patients have exaggerated deep tendon reflexes on the affected side. Later the limb is neglected and patients are often observed to ignore a functionless hand held on their lap which is devoid of any spontaneous movement.

7.2.3 Autonomic disturbance

In the acute stage of CRPS there is usually distal oedema in the affected limb and the skin is warm, red, and glossy. Some months later the limb becomes cold with mottled blue skin (Fig. 7.1). These changes are due to changes in regulation of peripheral perfusion. A minority of cases never exhibit the warm phase. The temperature difference between affected and normal limb is usually more than 1°C, although the magnitude and direction of this difference will vary according to environment. The specificity of the temperature change is high for diagnosis of CRPS, although sensitivity is only 32% under resting conditions. Sudomotor abnormality ranges from hyperhydrosis through to bone-dry skin.

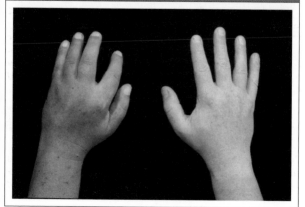

Fig 7.1 Early features of CRPS – note swelling and dusky appearance in left hand

7.2.4 **Trophic changes**

In the initial stages of CRPS there is increased hair and nail growth, while later this situation reverses with loss of skin features including hair. Eventually muscle atrophy and fixed contractures can occur.

7.2.5 **Natural history**

Previously three sequential stages of CRPS were described: an early acute phase resembling inflammation, an intermediate dystrophic phase, and a late atrophic stage, typified by loss of function, severe trophic features, and contracture. However, many patients do not follow this progression and the existence of sequential phases of CRPS is no longer recognized as useful in the diagnosis or management of CRPS. Indeed, some patients exhibit decreased skin temperature from the outset; this form of CRPS is associated with a poor prognosis, including ulceration and infection sometimes requiring amputation.

There is proximal spread from the original area affected in a contiguous manner in most cases, while in 70% symptoms and signs may appear in independent non-contiguous sites. Rarely, symptoms and signs will appear in the opposite limb as a mirror image of the original.

7.3 **Diagnosis**

CRPS is primarily a clinical diagnosis and the condition is probably overdiagnosed. More robust diagnostic criteria with high specificity but lower sensitivity have been proposed for research purposes (Box 7.2). There is no confirmatory diagnostic test for CRPS although other differential diagnoses may need to be excluded with appropriate investigations. Among the most useful investigations to support the diagnosis of CRPS are:

- plain radiology – osteoporotic change is common after the first few weeks
- three-phase bone scintigram – a three-phase bone scan with Technetium-99m will show increased uptake in later stages of the condition
- MRI – this will show widespread oedema in deep connective tissue, muscle, and peri-articular tissue
- Thermography – this will demonstrate any temperature difference between affected and normal limbs.

Box 7.2 Research criteria for diagnosis of CRPS

- Continuing pain disproportionate to inciting event
- At least one symptom from each of the following four categories:
  - sensory (hyperasthesia)
  - vasomotor (temperature asymmetry, skin colour change, or asymmetry)
  - sudomotor (oedema, sweating change, or asymmetry)
  - motor/trophic (reduced range of motion, weakness, tremor dystonia/nail, hair, skin changes)
- Must display at least one sign in two or more of the following categories:
  - sensory (hyperalgesia, allodynia)
  - vasomotor (temperature asymmetry, skin colour change, or asymmetry)
  - sudomotor (oedema, sweating change, or asymmetry)
  - motor/trophic (reduced range of motion, weakness, tremor dystonia/nail, hair, skin changes)

7.4 Pathophysiology

7.4.1 Overview

It seems most likely that CRPS is a systemic disease involving both the central and peripheral nervous system in susceptible individuals. In addition, the clinical course of CRPS is so variable that it is likely that there is no single mechanism involved and indeed there is some ongoing debate regarding the existence of CRPS as a single entity. Several mechanisms are thought to be relevant and are not necessarily specific to CRPS. The pathophysiology is clearly multifactorial and the exact nature of the initiating event may be relatively unimportant.

7.4.2 Regional or neurogenic inflammation

The acute stage of CRPS resembles acute inflammation yet several studies have failed to show typical inflammation in peripheral tissues. However, primary nociceptive afferent activation by cytokines released following trauma results in retrograde release of neuropeptides in the periphery, including substance P and calcitonin gene-related peptide. This process of neurogenic inflammation may produce the inflammatory-like features of CRPS, including increased skin temperature, oedema, and the trophic changes.

7.4.3 Sympathetic nervous system

There is considerable evidence suggesting that the sympathetic nervous system has a role in chronic neuropathic inflammatory pain states (Box 7.3). Following the initial skin temperature increase due to neurogenic inflammation, there is evidence of central sympathetic dysfunction manifest as limb temperature decrease with increased sweating. Initially, sympathetic noradrenergic control of blood vessels is reduced, producing vasodilation, and subsequently it is thought that the denervated blood vessels develop an increased sensitivity to catecholamine, resulting in vasoconstriction. There may be additional central failure of sympathetic control of vasoconstriction. There is evidence that in CRPS functional adrenoceptors are expressed on primary nociceptive afferents because subcutaneous injection of norepinephrine is painful while sympathetic blockade relieves pain.

The exact role of the sympathetic nervous system in CRPS remains controversial and it seems likely that pain due to sympathetic dysfunction – termed 'sympathetically maintained pain' (SMP) – overlaps with CRPS but is also relevant in other types neuropathic pain, while in many cases of CRPS, SMP is not relevant.

7.4.4 Central neuroplasticity

Patients with CRPS often report numbness and hyperalgesia in a neurological distribution outside that of the original injury, sometimes extending to a hemisensory impairment. These changes reverse if CRPS pain is relieved. This implies central nervous system plasticity at spinal or supraspinal level and there is evidence for both from studies using positron emission tomography and magneto-encephalography (MEG). MEG studies have demonstrated cortical reorganization of hand representation in patients with CRPS, which reverses with effective analgesia (Fig. 7.2) (see Chapter 2). Similar changes in cortical representation are observed in other neuropathic pain conditions, for example phantom limb pain.

Box 7.3 Supportive evidence for sympathetic system involvement in chronic neuropathic pain

- Increase in number of adrenoceptors in skin
- Expression of adrenoceptors in peripheral sensory afferents
- Topical α_2-adrenoceptor agonists decrease pain in the affected region (by pre-synaptic decrease in norepinephrine release)
- Sympathectomy reduces pain in some cases
- Stress or sympathetic stimulation increases pain

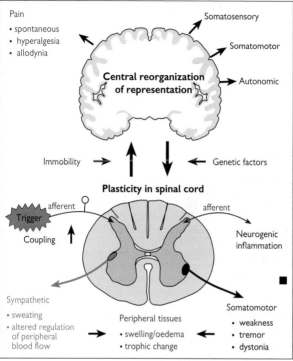

Figure 7.2 Sensory, motor and autonomic changes in CRPS type I. Changes are triggered by nociceptive afferent input. Afferent neurons may become sensitized to catecholamine by receptor expression or coupling to sympathetic efferents. CRPS is maintained by reorganization within the spinal cord resulting in retrograde neurogenic inflammation. Reorganization in higher centres results in pain, motor changes, and modified autonomic output.

7.4.5 Immobility

There is experimental evidence that prolonged immobilization can lead to changes similar to CRPS without the need for an injury or noxious event. The magnitude of the changes from such experimental immobilization is less than in clinical CRPS, suggesting that this mechanism is only contributory.

7.4.6 Genetic factors

An association with HLA-DR13 and HLA-DQ1 in patients with CRPS has been reported, suggesting a genetic susceptibility to CRPS. This might explain why only a few patients subject to a given trauma go on to develop CRPS.

7.4.7 **Psychological factors**

No specific psychological factors have been identified that predispose to CRPS, although secondary depression is common.

7.5 **Treatment**

There is no specific treatment for CRPS, perhaps because of the limited understanding of the underlying mechanisms. The management aims of type I and type II CRPS are similar and focus on the relief of pain and the restoration of function.

7.5.1 **Physical therapy**

It is suggested that restoration of function to the affected limb reduces pain and improves prognosis. Physiotherapy is the standard initial treatment for CRPS, using progressive desensitization and mobilization techniques, although progress may be limited by severe pain requiring additional treatment. It is important that active physical therapy is used and not the passive movement of an anaesthetized limb.

More specialized techniques have been used in CRPS, such as motor imagery training. This consists of sequential periods of hand laterality recognition, imagined movements, and lastly mirror movements. This technique has been shown to improve the symptoms of CRPS compared to passive mobilization. It is thought that the active nature of the treatment corrects inappropriate cortical remapping and thus it might be considered a mechanism-based treatment approach.

7.5.2 **Medication**

Non-steroidal anti-inflammatory drugs, opioids, and most co-analgesics have been used in the management of CRPS, using standard principles for neuropathic pain, with variable success. The oral route is usual although occasionally opioids and co-analgesics, especially the α_2 adrenergic antagonist clonidine, are delivered intrathecally. Calcitonin has been used with mixed results in CRPS.

7.5.3 **Sympathetic nervous system blockade**

Sympathetic interventions have been a traditional treatment for RSD for several decades because of early reports of efficacy. The sympathetic nervous system may be inhibited peripherally by means of intravenous regional sympathetic blockade comprising the injection of guanethidine (or bretylium) and local anaesthetic distal to a limb tourniquet. The guanethidine acts by temporarily displacing norepinephrine from adrenergic nerve endings. More proximal sympathetic blockade can be achieved with thoracic sympathectomy or stellate ganglion block for the upper limb and lumbar sympathectomy for the lower limb, temporarily using local anaesthetic or more permanently with neurolytic agents. Recently there has been an appreciation that sympathetic blockade is of limited value in the management of CRPS.

7.5.4 Somatic nerve blocks

Somatic local anaesthetic nerve blocks are used to facilitate physio-therapy and rehabilitation in CRPS by providing pain relief. Although there are no controlled trials there are numerous reports of continuous peripheral nerve blocks having been used in the management of CRPS. Commonly used blocks include continuous brachial plexus block and lumbar plexus blockade.

7.5.5 Amputation

Amputation remains a therapeutic option in severe CRPS; it is rarely recommended by clinicians but is often suggested by patients. High-quality evidence of effectiveness is lacking and amputation is certainly not a guaranteed solution for CRPS. The risk of long-term complications, including persisting pain and phantom pain, is real.

7.5.6 Neuromodulation

Neuromodulation involves the modification of pain transmission using non-destructive methods, the most common being high-frequency electrical stimulation. Transcutaneous electrical nerve stimulation (TENS; see Chapter 13) is commonly employed in the early management of CRPS, although the evidence of effectiveness is equivocal. The more invasive and expensive option of spinal cord stimulation (SCS; see Chapter 14), using an implanted epidural elec-trode stimulating system, has been demonstrated to have a modest beneficial effect in CRPS when combined with physical therapy. Minor technical problems are relatively common and SCS is usually a late treatment option.

7.5.7 Free radical scavengers

The demonstration of peripheral inflammatory mediators in CRPS has resulted in the use of free radical scavengers in an attempt to reduce the tissue-damaging effects of inflammation. Topical dimethyl-sulfoxide has been found to be effective for pain relief in warm CRPS, while systemic N-acetyl cysteine is effective in cold CRPS. Neither agent is in common use.

7.5.8 Prevention of CRPS following surgery

The development of CRPS as a complication of surgery is unpredict-able and so prevention is difficult, but it is recommended to avoid surgery on a limb currently affected by CRPS to avoid aggravation of the symptoms. Regional anaesthetic techniques are suggested to reduce the incidence and recurrence of CRPS, especially if sympa-thetic blockade is achieved. The use of free radical scavengers and various adrenergic blockers, for example ketanserin, have been suggested but evidence of effectiveness is limited. In general, effective multimodal peri-operative analgesia is probably the most effective way to guard against the development of CRPS.

Key references

Birklein, F. (2005). Complex regional pain syndrome. *J. Neurol.*, **252**, 131–8.

Janig, W. and Baron, R. (2003). Complex regional pain syndrome: mystery explained. *Lancet Neurology*, **2**, 687–91.

Ochoa, J.L. (1999). Truths, errors and lies around 'reflex sympathetic dystrophy' and complex regional pain syndrome. *J. Neurol.*, **246**, 875–9.

Raja, S.N. and Grabow, T.S. (2002). Complex regional pain syndrome I (reflex sympathetic dystrophy). *Anesthesiology*, **96**, 1254–60.

Stanton-Hicks, M., Janig, W., Hassenbusch, S., Haddox, J.D., Boas, R., Wilson, P. (1995). Reflex sympathetic dystrophy: changing concepts and taxonomy. *Pain*, **63**, 127–33.

Chapter 8

Cancer neuropathic pain

Fliss E. Murtagh and Irene J. Higginson

> ### Key points
> - Around a third of cancer pains may have a neuropathic component and mixed pathology is more usual than 'pure' neuropathic pain.
> - Compression and infiltration of nerves by tumour are the most common causes.
> - Treatment-induced damage (chemotherapy-induced neuropathy, radiation plexitis, surgical trauma) and paraneoplastic syndromes are less common causes.
> - Cancer patients are generally older and frailer than other chronic pain patients and may be more vulnerable to adverse drug effects.
> - First-line treatment with opioids is usual in this context but co-analgesics are almost certainly needed in addition.

8.1 Epidemiology

8.1.1 Limitations of existing studies

A recent systematic review on the epidemiology of cancer pain found that most studies of cancer pain prevalence do not categorize according to pathophysiology. That is, they do not specifically identify neuropathic pain. A review of pain in lung cancer (one of the commonest cancers to cause pain) similarly found that the causes or types of pain were infrequently described in the literature. Of 32 epidemiological pain studies identified, just four were classified by underlying cause of the pain and four by pathophysiological subtype.

8.1.2 Prevalence of cancer neuropathic pain

Despite these limitations, some conclusions can be drawn about the prevalence of cancer neuropathic pain. A prospective study of 2266 cancer patients referred to a pain service identified neuropathic pain in 34%, with over two-thirds of these pains directly caused by the cancer, and one in seven related to cancer treatment. An international survey of cancer pain in 1095 patients suggests that up to 40%

of cancer pain may have a neuropathic component. This comprises 23% with a combination of somatic and neuropathic pain, 5% with a combination of somatic, visceral, and neuropathic pain, 4% combined visceral and neuropathic in origin, and only 8% purely neuropathic. Both of these studies may overestimate the prevalence of neuropathic pain because the study populations were selected groups: those referred to a pain service and consecutive patients identified by clinicians with an interest in cancer pain, respectively. Neuropathic pain is reported to occur in 25–32% of lung cancer patients, although again these figures may reflect a somewhat higher prevalence than in cancer patients overall, because of greater frequency of malignant invasion of neurological structures and of neurological damage from anti-neoplastic treatment in lung, as compared with other, cancers. Overall, one-third of cancer pains may have a neuropathic component, and mixed pathophysiology is much more frequent than 'pure' neuropathic pain.

8.1.3 Types of nerve damage

One detailed study of cancer neuropathic pain suggests that 79% of cases result from nerve compression, 16% from nerve injury, and 5% are sympathetically mediated. There is some indication that reversible nerve compression may eventually progress to irreversible nerve injury, and that nerve injury pain may itself be more difficult to treat than nerve compression pain. Sympathetically mediated pain is particularly challenging to manage, and may be better classed as a type of complex regional pain syndrome. The latter includes (but is not confined to) sympathetically mediated pain. Categorizing pain in this more detailed way is difficult, both in clinical and research contexts, and this evidence should therefore be interpreted with caution.

8.2 Clinical presentation

8.2.1 Direct tumour infiltration of peripheral nerves

This most commonly occurs with rib metastases, or with paravertebral or retroperitoneal metastases. Presentation is directly related to the exact nerve or nerves involved, and usually can be relatively easily related to known spread of the cancer, as long as suspicion of metastatic spread to the site concerned is high (see Box 8.1 for causes of cancer neuropathic pain).

8.2.2 Tumour infiltration of plexi

Cervical plexopathy is commonly due to head and neck tumours or cervical lymph node metastases. Pain may occur in the pre-auricular, post-auricular, or anterior neck, and an associated ipsilateral Horner's syndrome or hemidiaphragmatic paralysis should be sought.

Box 8.1 Likely causes of cancer neuropathic pain

Predominantly acute pain

- Painful peripheral neuropathy due to chemotherapy toxicity (most commonly from vinca alkaloids, platinum compounds, or taxanes)
- Acute radiation-induced plexopathy or myelopathy

Predominantly chronic pain

- *Direct tumour infiltration of a peripheral nerve* – most commonly from paravertebral or retroperitoneal spread, or from rib metastases
- *Tumour infiltration of a nerve plexus* – cervical plexopathy is most common in primary head and neck tumours or metastases to the neck, brachial plexopathy is most common in lymphoma, breast, or lung cancer, and lumbosacral plexopathy is most often seen with pelvic tumours
- *Radiculopathy* – due to tumour spread to involve dorsal spinal nerve roots, most often from epidural tumour mass or leptomeningeal metastases
- *Painful peripheral neuropathy* – may be due to direct tumour spread, chemotherapy toxicity, metabolic causes such as diabetes or renal or hepatic dysfunction, nutritional deficiencies, or paraneoplastic syndromes
- *Post-surgical pain syndromes* – post-mastectomy, post-thoracotomy, post-radical neck dissection, and phantom limb pain are the commonest examples
- *Post radiation pain syndromes* – these are uncommon and other causes of pain, such as recurrent tumour, should be considered first

Brachial plexopathies occur usually as a result of axillary lymph node metastases in breast cancer or lymphoma, or because of direct extension of an apical lung cancer: Pancoast's tumour. They may present with upper plexus involvement (C5 and 6) or lower plexus involvement (C7, 8, and T1). In Pancoast's tumour, when there is direct extension from the lung apex, it is usually the lower plexus which is involved; pain often precedes neurological deficit and occurs particularly around the elbow, in the medial forearm, and fourth and fifth fingers.

Lumbosacral plexopathies are most often related to colorectal or cervical carcinomas, lymphomas, or metastases from breast cancer. Again, pain is often the first symptom, before any neurological deficit develops. Autonomic dysfunction is common, and motor and sensory deficits tend to occur subsequently. Pain presentation varies very much according to the part of the lumbosacral plexus involved, and may vary from pain in the back, low abdomen, flanks, and anterolateral thigh (upper plexus) to pain in the perineum, buttocks, and postero-lateral leg (lower plexus). Careful evaluation of lumbar and sacral neurological function is important, and deficits at multiple levels are usual.

8.2.3 Radiculopathies

Nerve damage to the dorsal spinal roots gives rise to radiculopathies. In cancer patients, this is most often caused by epidural tumour mass or leptomeningeal metastases. With epidural tumour mass, patients present with dermatomal pain in the affected territory; this tends to be unilateral in cervical and lumbosacral regions, and bilateral in the thorax. The pain is typically exacerbated by coughing or sneezing. Any presentation of this nature should lead to urgent consideration and investigation of associated spinal cord compression. Leptomeningeal metastases are less common, and may produce a variety of multifocal neurological symptoms and signs, including generalized headache and radicular pain in buttocks or lower back.

8.2.4 Painful peripheral neuropathy

The chemotherapeutic drugs associated with painful neuropathies are the vinca alkaloids (vinblastine, vincristine, vindesine, vinorelbine), platinum compounds (carboplatin, cisplatin, oxaliplatin), the taxanes (docetaxel and paclitaxel), procarbazine, and altretamine. Most of these agents, at usual doses, only infrequently cause painful neuropathies, but vincristine, vinorelbine, and cisplatin are more commonly problematic. Presentation is usually of painful or 'burning' hands or feet, with allodynia, hyperalgesia, or parasthesiae. A variety of sensory, motor, or autonomic deficits may be associated, and reduced tendon reflexes are common. Vinblastine and vincristine have also occasionally been linked to neuropathic jaw pain.

After discontinuation of the drug, symptoms usually subside slowly, although they may take several months to do so. Neuropathies associated with cisplatin may be more persistent. Thalidomide, although not a chemotherapeutic agent, is increasingly used in cancer patients, and may also cause painful peripheral neuropathy, usually reversible on stopping treatment.

8.2.5 Paraneoplastic syndromes

Paraneoplastic syndromes are themselves rare, occurring in just 6% of all cancer patients. Paraneoplastic sensory or sensorimotor neuropathies causing neuropathic pain are even less common, but are recognized most often in association with small-cell lung cancer, breast cancer, gynaecological malignancies, and myeloma. Patients usually present with an asymmetrical painful sensory or mixed sensorimotor neuropathy, but there is wide variation in both presentation and subsequent course. Metabolic or nutritional deficiencies may be a more likely cause of sensory neuropathies in cancer patients than paraneoplastic syndromes, and these should always be considered and excluded.

8.2.6 Post-surgical neuropathic pain

Neuropathic pain may also present following surgery; the commonest presentations are after mastectomy with axillary node dissection, post radical neck dissection, after thoracotomy, and phantom limb pain following amputation.

8.3 Assessment

8.3.1 Patient factors

A number of patient factors tend to make assessment and subsequent management of cancer neuropathic pain more challenging. These include:

- the generally older age of cancer patients
- the greater frailty and increased co-morbidity associated with older age
- the possible involvement of other organ systems in patients with advanced metastatic cancer (especially hepatic and renal impairment)
- the high frequency of cognitive impairment in patients with advanced cancer.

8.3.2 Identifying cancer neuropathic pain

As in non-cancer neuropathic pain, there is no single symptom or sign pathognomonic of cancer neuropathic pain. The infrequency of 'pure' neuropathic pain, and the fact that pain mechanisms are often mixed in cancer patients, means that it is particularly hard to achieve consistency in assessment. There is less agreement between independent assessors in the context of neuropathic pain compared to nociceptive pain, and it is often challenging to identify specific mechanisms and causes of pain in the individual patient. With cancer progression, different mechanisms may also change over time and the relationship between symptoms, signs, and mechanisms is unclear. It is best therefore to maintain a low threshold of suspicion for neuropathic pain, and actively seek out any features suggestive of neuropathic pain if:

- any pain in a cancer patient is persistent or severe
- any pain is particularly intense or distressing in quality
- any pain does not respond to standard approaches
- the known anatomical location of disease suggests a neuropathic component or pain from nerve compression or injury is likely
- treatment of the cancer has included one of the examples identified in Box 8.1.

Table 8.1 Important features of assessment in cancer neuropathic pain	
Symptom or sign	**Identify**
Pain	For both spontaneous and evoked pain: • location and radiation • pattern (onset, timing, and duration) • quality • severity or intensity • triggers (for evoked pain)
Sensory symptoms	Abnormal sensations (crawling, prickling, itching, or tingling) Numbness
Sensory signs	Sensory loss Colour changes Allodynia (pain from normally non-noxious stimuli) Hyperalgesia (increased sensitivity to normally painful stimuli)
Motor symptoms and signs	Motor symptoms and signs are often present but can be subtle
Other considerations	**Explore**
Co-morbidity	Concurrent illness, and impact of metastatic disease on other systems
Prognosis	Expected course of disease – consider whether suspected cause of neuropathic pain is likely to worsen
Impact on quality of life	Overall function and disability Psychological and emotional effects Family impact

Assessment tools may be helpful. In particular, the Leeds Assessment of Neuropathic Symptoms and Signs scale is simple and has been shown to be suitable for assessing neuropathic pain in cancer patients, although changes in skin appearance or colour may be less useful as an indicator of neuropathic pain in cancer patients.

8.3.3 Other considerations

In the history, it is important to identify co-morbidity, especially diabetes mellitus, and previous liver or renal disease, since these may increase the likelihood of painful peripheral neuropathy. A careful history of the cancer is also crucial, including results of any staging investigations, in order to clarify the known or suspected location of the primary tumour and any direct or secondary spread. Also important are the full details of any treatment received, including radiotherapy, chemotherapy (exact chemotherapeutic agents and doses used), and any surgical treatment. A detailed history of the pain, associated symptoms, and the impact on the patient and family is then required, with particular attention to the features identified in Table 8.1.

8.4 **Treatment**

8.4.1 **General approaches**

Management of cancer-related neuropathic pain is often challenging and a number of different therapeutic options may be required, either concurrently or sequentially. Pain brings its own psychological costs to the patient, but the additional psychological impact of prolonged titration and adjustment of medication, and changes in therapeutic approach, should not be underestimated. Clear and consistent explanation of proposed management to patient and family at each stage can make a major difference in lessening this impact and maintaining levels of trust between the patient and professionals.

In general, pharmacological management of cancer neuropathic pain draws heavily on evidence from studies in non-cancer conditions, and limited work has been done in patients with cancer neuropathic pain. However, there are some specific issues in cancer neuropathic pain which will be highlighted here.

8.4.2 **Opioids**

While there is good evidence that opioids are effective in non-cancer neuropathic pain, there is much less evidence in cancer neuropathic pain. What evidence there is suggests that the overall responsiveness of cancer neuropathic pain to opioids is less than for cancer nociceptive pain. However, the response of any individual patient cannot be predicted, and higher doses may be effective. A trial of opioid is therefore recommended first-line, but with the expectation that careful titration of doses upwards to effect or until intolerable side-effects intervene may be required. Co-analgesics are almost certainly needed alongside opioids (Box 8.2).

There is insufficient evidence to suggest that any one opioid has specific advantages over another. Given the absence of data, including lack of comparative studies and the wide individual variability in response to different opioids, a low threshold for switch to an alternative opioid is suggested. Combining two opioids may, in future, improve the management of cancer neuropathic pain, but research is needed to indicate which opioids or doses might be beneficial.

> **Box 8.2 Steps in the use of opioid analgesia in cancer neuropathic pain**
>
> - Optimize the opioid regimen (no one opioid can be recommended above another).
> - Titrate upwards until effect or intolerable side-effects.
> - Maximally manage side-effects to allow for further titration if possible.
> - Ensure all appropriate non-pharmacological interventions have been considered.
> - If unacceptable opioid side-effects persist without adequate analgesic effect, consider:
>   - adjuvant analgesics
>   - switching to an alternative opioid.

8.4.3 Antidepressants

Limited evaluation of tricyclic antidepressants has taken place in cancer neuropathic pain. However, existing evidence combined with extensive clinical experience suggests tricyclics are effective in this context. Their main disadvantage is frequent antimuscarinic side-effects, including cardiotoxicity, hypotension, and confusion, which are problematic in the elderly cancer patient or those with cardiac co-morbidity. Newer antidepressants such as venlafaxine may be better tolerated but show limited effectiveness.

8.4.4 Anti-epileptics

There is considerable evidence to support the use of gabapentin in non-cancer neuropathic pain, and this has been extrapolated by clinicians to apply to cancer patients. One study has provided early evidence that gabapentin may be beneficial to patients with cancer neuropathic pain, but the side-effects of dizziness and sedation may limit dose titration because patients are frailer. In the light of possible synergistic effects between morphine and gabapentin, concurrent reduction of opioid doses may be needed.

Key references

Bennett, M.I. (2005). Gabapentin significantly improves analgesia in people receiving opioids for neuropathic cancer pain. *Cancer Treat. Rev.*, **31** (1), 58–62. [Commentary on: Caraceni, A., Zecca, E., Bonezzi, C., Arcuri, E., Yaya Tur R., Maltoni, M. (2004). Gabapentin for neuropathic cancer pain: a randomized controlled trial for the Gabapentin Cancer Pain Study Group. *J. Clin. Oncol.*, **22**, 2909–17.]

Caraceni, A., and Portenoy, R.K. (1999). An international survey of cancer pain characteristics and syndromes. IASP Task Force on Cancer Pain. International Association for the Study of Pain. *Pain*, **82** (3), 263–74.

Cherny, N.I., Thaler, H.T., Friedlander-Klar, H., Lapin, J., Foley, K.M., Houde, R., *et al.* (1994). Opioid responsiveness of cancer pain syndromes caused by neuropathic or nociceptive mechanisms: a combined analysis of controlled, single-dose studies. *Neurology*, **44** (5), 857–61.

Goudas, L.C., Bloch, R., Gialeli-Goudas, M., Lau, J., and Carr D.B. (2005). The epidemiology of cancer pain. *Cancer Invest*, **23** (2), 182–90.

Grond, S., Zech, D., Diefenbach, C., Radbruch, L., and Lehmann, K.A. (1996). Assessment of cancer pain: a prospective evaluation in 2266 cancer patients referred to a pain service. *Pain*, **64** (1), 107–14.

Potter, J., and Higginson, I.J. (2004). Pain experienced by lung cancer patients: a review of prevalence, causes and pathophysiology. *Lung Cancer*, **43** (3), 247–57.

Potter, J., Higginson, I.J., Scadding, J.W., and Quigley, C. (2003). Identifying neuropathic pain in patients with head and neck cancer: use of the Leeds Assessment of Neuropathic Symptoms and Signs scale. *J. Roy. Soc. Med.*, **96** (8), 379–83.

Part 2

Treatment

Chapter 9

Antidepressants and anti-epileptics for neuropathic pain

Henry J. McQuay and Philip Wiffen

> ### Key points
>
> - Antidepressants and anti-epileptics are well-established treatments for neuropathic pain.
> - Clinical trial evidence can be limited in both scope of neuropathic pain conditions studied and duration of treatment. This leaves prescribers to extrapolate evidence to other conditions, and without information on longer-term effects.
> - Lack of head-to-head comparisons results in the use of indirect evidence such as NNTs, but the sample size used to derive NNT values is equally important.
> - Although tricyclics appear more effective than other classes of antidepressants, this needs to be balanced against higher incidence of adverse effects.
> - League tables suggest that the character of the neuropathic pain, whether it be burning or shooting, does not determine its responsiveness to either of the drug classes.

9.1 Introduction

9.1.1 Background to antidepressants and anti-epileptics

The first reports of anti-epileptic efficacy in trigeminal neuralgia go back nearly fifty years, and tricyclic antidepressant efficacy was also shown in a variety of pain syndromes decades ago. Our concern now is not whether antidepressants and anti-epileptics work in neuropathic pain, although we still have to show that for any new drugs that come along, but how well do the different drugs within the antidepressant and anti-epileptic categories work compared with each other, and indeed how well do antidepressants work compared with anti-epileptics? The other side of the coin is the relative adverse effect burden within and between the two drug classes. Exactly how effective the two drug classes are, and at what cost in adverse effects, remains a focus of attention for clinicians, researchers, and the patients themselves.

9.1.2 Antidepressant pharmacology

Tricyclic antidepressants (TCAs) such as amitriptyline and imipramine have a multimodal mechanism of action. They inhibit pre-synaptic uptake of serotonin and noradrenaline, interact with sodium and calcium ion channels, and block some post-synaptic histamine and muscarinic receptors. Tricyclics generally show non-linear pharmacokinetics, meaning that there is no linear relationship between drug dose and steady state serum concentration. For example, a 30-fold difference in serum concentrations has been observed on the same TCA dose in different patients. This can also result in significantly higher serum concentrations (and clinical effects) despite small dose changes, and vice versa. Dry mouth, drowsiness, and postural hypotension are the most frequent adverse effects and are often more pronounced in the elderly. In general, sub-antidepressant doses of TCAs can produce analgesic benefit; the usual starting dose of amitriptyline is 25mg daily, titrated to a mean of around 75mg.

More selective antidepressants include selective serotonin reuptake inhibitors (SSRIs) such as paroxetine and fluoxetine, and balanced serotonin noradrenaline reuptake inhibitors (SNRIs) such as venlafaxine and the more potent duloxetine (the latter is licensed for painful diabetic neuropathy). Both these drug classes have virtually no blocking effects on post-synaptic receptors or ion channels, leading to fewer side-effects. A current debate is to what extent the multimodal action of TCAs contributes to their apparent superiority, as well as greater adverse effects, compared with SSRIs and SNRIs in treating neuropathic pain.

9.1.3 Anti-epileptic pharmacology

The mechanism of action of older anti-epileptic drugs, such as phenytoin and carbamazepine, was thought to occur via blockade of voltage-dependent sodium channels. However, recent work suggests that carbamazepine may in fact have additional actions via serotonergic pathways (which is not surprising as it is structurally very similar to TCAs). Newer anti-epileptics, such as gapapentin, pregabalin, and lamotrigine, have actions on various receptors, including the $\alpha_2\delta$ sub-unit of voltage-dependent calcium channels and modulation of GABA synthesis, release, and metabolism. Adverse effects are similar for all anti-epileptics and those most frequently reported are drowsiness, fatigue, and ataxia. Longer-term adverse effects are not always apparent in clinical trials of short duration, and weight gain associated with gabapentin is an example of this. Doses of anti-epileptics used to treat neuropathic pain are generally similar to those used in epilepsy. (See also Chapter 10 for parenteral use of anti-epileptic drugs.)

9.2 Clinical trial evidence

9.2.1 Issues of scope

The focus on the relative efficacy and adverse effect rates of the two drug classes has made us think more about neuropathic pain in general, and about the trials, their conduct, and outcomes used in reporting them. A simple example of the wider issues is whether or not you include fibromyalgia as a neuropathic pain symptom. It responds to the same drug classes but is unlike other neuropathic pain syndromes in that there is no demonstrable nervous system dysfunction.

Most of the trials from which the information below was drawn were done in post-herpetic neuralgia (PHN) and painful diabetic neuropathy (PDN). These two conditions are relatively easy to diagnose and have therefore become the test-bed of choice for testing drug efficacy in neuropathic pain. But most neuropathic pain is not PHN or PDN. Historically, drug remedies for PHN and PDN have been effective in other neuropathic pain syndromes, but we do not know if negative results in PHN and PDN are predictive of lack of efficacy in other neuropathic pain syndromes. Much of our prescribing for neuropathic pain involves this kind of extrapolation from results in other, different, pain syndromes.

9.2.2 Issues of duration

For the trials themselves one of the major questions is how long – weeks or months – should the drug be studied for us to be certain of its efficacy. Many neuropathic pain syndromes may need medication for years, so that issues of efficacy and safety over the longer term are important to patients and prescribers. Most of the trials, however, are of less than eight weeks' duration, and it is only for the very recently introduced drugs that we have information for up to three months of treatment. Even this is limited in relation to the duration of the condition. We just do not know the proportion of patients in whom initial drug efficacy subsequently wanes and over what period any such waning occurs. Neither do we know the corollary, the proportion in whom initial drug efficacy is maintained without dose escalation for one or indeed five years.

Technically, neuropathic pain trials may be difficult trials to run because for many of the antidepressant and anti-epileptic drugs there has to be a titration to the optimal dose for maximal effect and minimal adverse effects, and trial designs necessarily become complicated to incorporate this titration. The alternative (using fixed doses of these drugs) risks underdosing some patients and overdosing others, as well as underestimating efficacy and overestimating adverse effects.

9.3 **Determining relative efficacy**

9.3.1 **Lack of head-to-head (direct) evidence**

There are surprisingly few head-to-head comparisons of antidepressants and anti-epileptics in neuropathic pain, and even fewer head-to-head comparisons either between different antidepressants or between different anti-epileptics. Indeed, the small numbers of patients studied in these conditions may come as a surprise. An example is that all the sweeping statements made about the lack of efficacy of SSRIs in neuropathic pain are based on the grand total of 80 patients studied in trials of good quality, and in one of those trials the SSRI did just as well as the tricyclic antidepressant. Perhaps the emergence of medical myths is in inverse proportion to the amount of data.

In the only modern head-to-head comparison, a small study of 19 patients who crossed over between gabapentin (up to 1800mg) and amitriptyline (up to 75mg) in painful diabetic neuropathy found that there was no significant difference in pain scores with the two drugs, or in global ratings of pain relief (52% with at least moderate pain relief during gabapentin and 67% during amitriptyline) ($P > 0.1$). Both treatments caused similar rates of adverse events.

9.3.2 **Using systematic review (indirect) evidence**

In the absence of head-to-head or direct comparisons of these drugs in neuropathic pain, how are we to arrive at an assessment of the relative efficacy and tolerability of the different drugs? Earlier reviews and the most recent updates have used systematic review techniques to gather the data from good-quality trials comparing anti-epileptics or antidepressants with placebo, the indirect method. The efficacy of the different drugs against placebo is then calculated and expressed as the number-needed-to-treat (NNT). The NNT values of the different drugs may then be compared to determine the relative efficacy of the different drugs.

An analogy might be that we want to know who is the quickest runner in the room. We could simply make everyone run 100 metres, competing with each other in one race, the direct method. This would be the head-to-head comparison. We could alternatively get each individual to run 100 metres against the clock and on their own. We could then compare the times to work out who was quickest. This latter indirect method is the equivalent of deriving the relative efficacy by comparing each drug's performance against placebo. To estimate the relative efficacy of anti-epileptics and antidepressants in neuropathic pain, we do not have a choice. We do not have direct comparisons, so we have to use an indirect method.

9.3.3 Limitations of indirect methods

These direct and indirect methods of assessing the efficacy of drugs used to manage neuropathic pain produce remarkably similar estimates, so one need not apologize for using the indirect technique. It is important, however, to be aware of the weaknesses, and of these by far the most significant is size. If the performance of the drug or even the drug class is based on a small number of patients studied, then the estimate of that performance should be treated with caution. An estimate of efficacy derived from 500 patients compared with placebo is likely to be a great deal more robust than one obtained on just 80 patients.

This sounds obvious and is obvious, but it is forgotten constantly, and casual mention of the NNT value for a particular treatment in neuropathic pain without reference to the size of the sample from which it was derived is misleading at the very least (see Chapter 16 for further discussion of NNT values). Fig.9.1 (taken from Finnerup et al, 2005) shows the range of NNT values in peripheral neuropathic pain for a number of antidepressant and anti-epileptic drugs. The diameter of the point estimate for each drug is proportional to the number of patients on whom the estimate is based, and the number is printed beside the estimate.

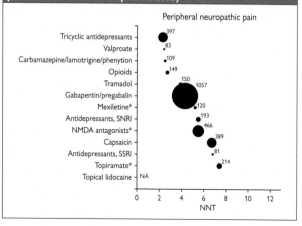

Fig 9.1 Number-needed-to-treat (NNT) values for different drug treatments in peripheral neuropathic pain (with permission from Finnerup et al. 2005)

9.3.4 **Comparing different antidepressant classes**

For tricyclic antidepressants, an NNT estimate of just over 2 means that roughly one patient in two treated with a tricyclic antidepressant for their peripheral neuropathic pain will achieve at least 50% pain relief. The other patient might have some relief, but not enough to take them past the 50% relief mark. The estimate is based on roughly 400 patients. These patients may have been on different antidepressants, and at different doses. The different doses should not be too much of a problem because the dose for each patient should have been the optimal dose. If we are hypercritical and insist on splitting the efficacy estimate into the individual tricyclic drugs, then we will have little data for most of the individual drugs.

The NNT estimate with SSRI antidepressants is over 6, meaning that just one patient in six treated with an SSRI antidepressant for their peripheral neuropathic pain will achieve at least 50% pain relief, much worse than for the TCAs. Again the other five patients on the SSRI might have had some relief, but did not achieve 50% relief. The estimate is based on just 81 patients, and is in stark contrast to the more than 1000 patients studied on gabapentin with an NNT estimate of just over 4. The smaller the point estimate in the figure, the less robust the estimate.

9.3.5 **The need for more clinical trials**

It has to be a concern that we have so little data on which to base important prescribing decisions. Using the antidepressants as an example, we would argue that SSRIs have not been adequately tested in neuropathic pain. The potential advantage of the lower adverse effect incidence with these drugs means perhaps that we need trials of adequate size and quality to check whether it really is true to say that SSRIs do not work in neuropathic pain. The number needed to harm (NNH) for trial withdrawal due to adverse effects of TCAs compared with placebo was estimated by Finnnerup *et al.* at 14.7 (10.2–25.2). In contrast there was no statistically significant difference between SSRI and placebo for withdrawal due to adverse effects.

Interestingly, the efficacy NNT values for the mixed SNRIs, tested in modern trials of high quality, are, at around 4, very similar to the NNTs for gabapentin, and, like SSRIs, the adverse effect profile of the SNRIs is better than TCAs, with no statistically significant difference for withdrawal due to adverse effects compared with placebo. It is also possible that the 'best buy' status of TCAs in the relative efficacy league table may be due to overestimation of benefit in older small trials, some of crossover design.

Against that interpretation, however, is the finding that in both painful polyneuropathy and post-herpetic neuralgia there is a trend towards better effect of balanced serotonin and noradrenaline reuptake inhibitors than of the mainly noradrenergic drugs. It will take fresh trials rather than meta-analysis to resolve the truth of the teaching of the past decades that the pharmacological 'shotgun' or multiple receptor action of the TCAs is more effective in neuropathic pain than the more selective or 'rifle' drugs.

9.4 **Using relative efficacy**

9.4.1 **League tables**

Diagnosing neuropathic pain is not difficult until people make it complicated. The combination of pain in an area of altered nervous system function, sometimes associated with pain on non-painful stimulus or excessive pain with a not very painful stimulus, and with a muted response to conventional analgesics, leads most clinicians to think of initiating treatment with antidepressant or anti-epileptic. The choices of which drug class to use for initial treatment, and which particular drug to use within that drug class, are where the league table of relative efficacy can help. The term 'league table' is used to mean a ranking of the NNT efficacy values of the different drugs, where the lowest value is best and the highest worst (Fig.9.1).

The league table is of course based on results from many patients, whereas you are treating an individual patient, and takes little or no account of the adverse effects which are so important for chronic therapy. Nonetheless we have to start somewhere, and the league table provides us with the probability of success and the extent of that success for the different drugs so that we can make more informed decisions.

9.4.2 **Treatment algorithm for antidepressants and anti-epileptics**

The algorithm produced by Finnerup et al. (Fig.9.2) is a practical example of where this process of meta-analysis can take us in the management of neuropathic pain. The algorithm attempts to encapsulate the evidence into a decision tree. The reality is that we lack the 'head-to-head' drug comparison studies necessary to put more flesh on the bones of the algorithm, and we lack understanding as to whether different mechanisms underlying various neuropathic pain syndromes mean that we should have a different algorithm for each condition. For instance, standard teaching used to be that one would use an antidepressant for a burning pain and an anti-epileptic for a shooting pain. There is little evidence to support this adage and indeed some evidence which goes against it, suggesting that the character of the pain, whether it be burning or shooting, does not determine its responsiveness to either of the drug classes.

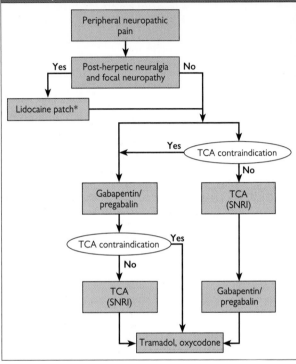

Fig 9.2 Algorithm for sequence of different drug treatments in peripheral neuropathic pain (with permission from Finnerup et al. 2005)

A thought-provoking paper from Denmark suggests that current methods of dividing neuropathic pain and thinking of different underlying mechanisms does not help in predicting response to the different drugs. Intriguingly, the patients who did not respond to imipramine (the test TCA) tended not to respond well to the second-line drug, the anti-epileptic gabapentin. For the moment it is one algorithm for all the different mechanisms underlying peripheral neuropathic pain.

Key references

Finnerup, N.B., Otto, M., McQuay, H.J., Jensen, T.S., and Sindrup, S.H. (2005). Algorithm for neuropathic pain treatment: an evidence-based proposal. *Pain*, **118**, 289–305.

Morello, C.M., Leckband, S.G., and Stoner, C.P. (1999). Randomized double-blind study comparing the efficacy of gabapentin with amitriptyline on diabetic peripheral neuropathy pain. *Arch. Intern. Med.*, **159**, 1931–7.

Rasmussen, P.V., Sindrup, S.H., Jensen, T.S., and Bach, F.W. (2004). Therapeutic outcome in neuropathic pain: relationship to evidence of nervous system lesion. *Eur. J. Neurol.*, **11**, 545–53.

Saarto, T. and Wiffen, P.J. (2005). Antidepressants for neuropathic pain. Cochrane Database of Systematic Reviews; CD005454.

Sindrup, S.H., Otto, M., Finnerup, N.B., and Jensen, T.S. (2005). Antidepressants in the treatment of neuropathic pain. *Basic Clin. Pharmacol. Toxicol.*, **96**, 399–409.

Wiffen, P., Collins, S., McQuay, H., Carroll, D., Jadad, A., and Moore, A. (2005). Anticonvulsant drugs for acute and chronic pain. Cochrane Database of Systematic Reviews; CD001133.

Wiffen, P.J., McQuay, H.J., Edwards, J.E., and Moore, R.A. (2005). Gabapentin for acute and chronic pain. Cochrane Database of Systematic Reviews; CD005452.

Wiffen, P.J., McQuay, H.J., and Moore, R.A. (2005). Carbamazepine for acute and chronic pain. Cochrane Database of Systematic Reviews; CD005451.

Chapter 10

Local anaesthetics and other pharmacological approaches

Gary McCleane

> ## Key points
>
> - While antidepressants, anti-epileptics, and opioids form the mainstay of neuropathic pain management, alternative approaches are needed because not all patients respond to these drugs and side-effects can limit their use in others.
> - Topically applied drugs such a lidocaine 5% patches and capsaicin cream can produce local analgesic effects, though lidocaine is better tolerated.
> - Baclofen and tizanadine are conventionally used as skeletal muscle relaxants but can be effective neuropathic pain agents.
> - The analgesic effects of cannabinoids have not been as significant as were initially expected.
> - Intravenous fosphenytoin and lidocaine are useful adjuncts for reducing acute flare-ups of neuropathic pain.

While the conventional pharmacological treatment of neuropathic pain revolves around the use of the opioid analgesics, tricyclic antidepressants, and anti-epileptic drugs, a variety of other pharmacological entities outside these groups are used successfully in some patients with neuropathic pain.

10.1 Topical agents

10.1.1 Role of topical agents

Many patients like the concept of applying medication to the site where discomfort is felt. Of course, in the case of neuropathic pain this may not actually be where the abnormal neural function that generates the pain is occurring. Nevertheless, there are some neuropathic pain conditions where the abnormal process is either peripherally located from the start, or where peripheral neural changes occur as a result of a more central neural dysfunction. In these cases, peripheral application of a variety of agents can produce pain relief.

When drugs are applied topically, the effect can be due to either a localized peripheral effect, to a more central effect consequent on systemic absorption of the drug, or a combination of both. This chapter concentrates on drugs with a predominantly peripheral effect. Examples of those with a transdermal application but with predominantly central effects, such as transdermal fentanyl and buprenorphine, are covered elsewhere (see Chapter 12).

10.1.2 **Lidocaine**

The numbing effect of local anaesthetics occurs because of the sodium channel-blocking effect of the local anaesthetic in question. This numbing effect is easily achieved by infiltration of the local anaesthetic into the skin. However, such use of a local anaesthetic is impractical in those suffering from neuropathic pain. Fortunately, a simple method of topical local anaesthetic deposition exists in the form of the lidocaine 5% patch. This is applied to the area over which the pain is experienced, with only a small proportion of lidocaine that is contained in the patch being absorbed through the skin. That which is absorbed is enough in some cases to provide pain relief. Because of the small amounts of lidocaine actually absorbed, systemic side-effects do not occur.

Lidocaine 5% patch has been well verified in the treatment of postherpetic neuralgia, but can also be a useful treatment in a wide variety of neuropathic and other pain conditions. Time to effect is measured in hours to a few days.

An added advantage of the lidocaine 5% patch is that it forms a physical barrier between the skin and, for example, clothing, which can reduce the discomfort of clothing rubbing against an area where allodynia, a common symptom of neuropathic pain, is experienced.

10.1.3 **Capsaicin**

Capsaicin, derived from the chilli pepper, has been used in medicinal practice for over 150 years. Repeated application results in absorption of capsaicin into peripheral nerves and axonal transport to the synaptic endings within the dorsal horn. Pain reduction is achieved by the propensity of capsaicin to inhibit the release of substance P from nerve endings and to reduce the density of epidermal nerve fibres. Because these effects are gradual and reversible, the time to effect can be at least two weeks and on occasions up to four weeks, and can occur only with repetitive and consistent application. Clearly it is only of potential value were the pain is of peripheral origin and covers a relatively small area. Capsaicin cream is commercially available in 0.025% and 0.075% concentrations.

The most common adverse effect associated with capsaicin application is a burning, tingling discomfort at the site of application along with mechanical and thermal allodynia. Usually these unpleasant effects reduce as time progresses, although application of capsaicin outside the area of normal application at any stage can cause a reappearance of these effects. This application discomfort not infrequently leads to a failure in compliance (Box 10.1).

Box 10.1 Strategies to minimize side-effects with capsaicin

- Apply in small volumes only.
- Use disposable gloves for application.
- Persist with application, if possible, as discomfort of application usually diminishes with time.
- Surround areas of application with petroleum jelly to prevent application outside the reference area.
- Pre-treatment with a topical local anaesthetic (e.g. EMLA, amethocaine gel) can minimize application discomfort.
- Addition of gylceryl trinitrate ointment to capsaicin cream reduces application discomfort and can enhance the analgesic effect of the capsaicin.

Occasionally sneezing can also occur, either in the patient or others living in close proximity, and usually occurs with over-application, drying of the cream on the skin, and the dust from this dried capsaicin being nasally inhaled. Caution should be used with capsaicin application to avoid application to moist areas (as this often exacerbates the discomfort associated with application) and that it is not accidentally applied to others, as in the case of a mother using the cream and then attending to a baby or child.

10.1.4 **Tricyclic antidepressants**

It is well accepted that oral tricyclic antidepressants can reduce neuropathic pain. This effect is achieved by virtue of a number of their modes of action:

- augmenting descending bulbo-spinal serotonergic inhibition
- augmenting descending bulbo-spinal noradrenergic inhibition
- an effect on NMDA (*N*-methyl D-aspartate) receptors
- an effect on opioid receptors
- sodium channel-blocking effects
- adenosine receptor-blocking effects

We know that adenosine receptors, sodium channels, and opioid receptors have a peripheral, as well as central, representation, and therefore their analgesic effect may be peripheral as well as central. Both animal and human studies confirm that topical application of tricyclic antidepressants can reduce neuropathic pain and that this effect is locally generated and not caused by systemic absorption. Time to effect is two to four weeks and side-effects are rare, providing application volumes and area of application are not excessive. Commercially, the tricyclic antidepressant doxepin is available as a 5% cream.

10.1.5 **Clonidine**

Clonidine, an α_2-adrenoreceptor agonist, is available in a patch formulation to enable transdermal administration. Two distinct effects can be achieved with transdermal clonidine. Firstly, a systemic effect which can alleviate neuropathic pain in a subset of patients with, for example, painful diabetic neuropathy. Secondly, it can reduce allodynia by a local action in some patients with sympathetically maintained pain.

10.2 **Oral agents**

10.2.1 **Mexiletine**

This oral, lidocaine-like, sodium channel-blocking anti-arrhythmic agent has been shown to have some effect in some patients with neuropathic pain. It has a narrow therapeutic index so use of effective dosages of mexiletine is not infrequently complicated by side-effects such as gastrointestinal upset and sedation.

10.2.2 **Baclofen**

Baclofen, a gamma amino butyric acid-B (GABA$_B$) agonist, is conventionally used as a skeletal muscle relaxant. However, it has been shown to reduce the pain associated with trigeminal neuralgia which is typified by intermittent flare-ups. Because of its fairly rapid onset of action, it can be used as an analgesic during these flare-ups. In most cases it is well tolerated and can be used with a starting dose of 10mg three times daily (decreased in the young, elderly, and infirm), increased up to a total of 60mg daily, if required.

10.2.3 **Tizanadine**

Again conventionally used as a skeletal muscle relaxant, tizanadine acts as an α_2-adrenoreceptor agonist. By virtue of this effect it can reduce neuropathic pain. Its principal side-effect is somnolence and therefore its use is particularly contemplated in the patient with neuropathic pain with secondary muscle spasm. The greater proportion of the daily dose is given at night to aid sleep.

10.2.4 **Cannabinoids**

Cannabinoids act both peripherally, via agonism at the specific cannabinoid receptors CB_1 and CB_2, and centrally. Much interest has focused on their use both as analgesics in neuropathic pain and as muscle relaxants. However, analysis of studies that examine the effect of the cannabinoids suggests that their analgesic effect in neuropathic pain is not as great as was initially suggested.

10.2.5 **$5HT_3$ antagonists**

The $5HT_3$ antagonist drugs are well established in the treatment of nausea and vomiting. They are now known to specifically block the neurokinin-1 (NK_1) expressing neurons in the dorsal horn of the spinal cord. These NK_1 expressing neurons are an important link in the spino-bulbo-cerebral transmission of pain signals and influence the descending control of dorsal horn function (see Chapter 2).

Use of a $5HT_3$ antagonist can therefore reduce certain types of pain and this includes neuropathic pain. They have a relatively benign side-effect profile with constipation and headache being the principal side-effects associated with sustained use. Members of the class include ondansetron, granisetron, dolasetron, and tropisetron.

10.2.6 **Cholecystokinin antagonists**

Cholecystokinin (CCK), originally described as a gut peptide, is now known to have central nervous system as well as gastrointestinal tract representation. The levels of this peptide in the central nervous system are increased by neural injury and sustained use of opioids, and it acts as an anti-opioid peptide. In animal pain models, administration of a CCK antagonist can not only enhance opioid-derived anti-nociception but also prevent and reverse established anti-nociceptive tolerance. To date, the human evidence merely suggests that the CCK antagonist proglumide enhances opioid-derived pain relief, with the question of its effects on opioid analgesic tolerance being unanswered.

10.3 **Parenteral agents**

10.3.1 **Need for parenteral agents**

While long-term pharmacological therapy of neuropathic pain is best achieved by use of topical or oral preparations, there are occasions when parenteral administration of medication is desirable:

• when the oral route of administration is unavailable (for example when severe vomiting is taking place)

- when a rapid titration of drug is needed during acute flare-ups of neuropathic pain
- when oral therapy is insufficient on its own to reduce acute pain
- when, as with intravenous lidocaine, phenytoin, and fosphenytoin, the duration of analgesic effect of the drug far outlives the plasma half-life of the drug.

10.3.2 **Lidocaine**

For over 50 years it has been known that the intravenous (IV) infusion of local anaesthetics can be associated with pain relief in a wide variety of pain conditions, including neuropathic pain. Since the introduction of lidocaine this effect has been confirmed on numerous occasions with this drug.

Both animal experimentation and human use suggests that the pain-relieving effect that can be apparent after IV lidocaine infusion can be of significantly greater duration than the half-life of the drug. Indeed, weeks of pain relief can follow IV lidocaine infusion. Despite the fear of potential cardiovascular side-effects, cardiac arrhythmia and evidence of any negative inotropic effect are very uncommon.

A number of unanswered questions remain about IV lidocaine use:

- the optimal dose administered
- the optimal infusion period
- whether a single infusion or repeated infusions achieve maximum effect
- the role of a test infusion of lidocaine at a lower dose than a formal infusion
- whether a positive response to IV lidocaine actually confirms that oral mexiletine has a greater chance of achieving pain relief.

Despite these questions, there is no doubt that IV lidocaine infusion represents a useful treatment of neuropathic pain. When it is effective, patients can reduce their concomitant analgesic consumption as well as potentially reducing other agents, such as tricyclic antidepressants and anti-epileptic drugs whose use is frequently associated with side-effects such as somnolence, weight gain, and effects on cognitive processes.

10.3.3 **Phenytoin**

It is of no surprise that the anti-epileptic drug phenytoin, known to have anti-neuropathic pain effects when used orally, can also reduce such pain when given parenterally (see also Chapter 9). However, caution with IV phenytoin use is needed as the parenteral formulations contain highly alkaline substances, and so any extravasation of the infused phenytoin can cause skin necrosis.

10.3.4 **Fosphenytoin**

Fosphenytoin is a water-soluble, ester pro-drug of phenytoin with a near normal pH. Consequently, the danger of skin necrosis is significantly less than with phenytoin. It shares the analgesic effect of phenytoin and as such is a safer, if more expensive, alternative to parenteral phenytoin.

10.3.5 **5HT$_3$ antagonists**

As mentioned above, the 5HT$_3$ antagonists can reduce pain associated with a variety of pain conditions, including that of neuropathic origin. By virtue of their lack of sedating effects and their general safety profile, IV 5HT$_3$ antagonists can be usefully administered when a rapid resolution of neuropathic pain is required.

10.3.6 **Adenosine**

Adenosine receptors have both peripheral and central nervous system representation and animal work suggests that these receptors have a function in nociceptive transmission. Isolated human reports suggest that IV infusion of adenosine can achieve sustained pain relief in some patients with refractory neuropathic pain.

10.4 **Using other pharmacological approaches in practice**

Not all patients with neuropathic pain can be successfully treated with tricyclics, anti-epileptics, or opioids. In further patients intolerable side-effects are apparent after use of drugs in these classes. It is therefore important to have alternatives. With some of the options listed in this chapter, a wealth of experience with their use exists. In others, such as the 5HT$_3$ antagonists and CCK antagonists, only time will tell if their use becomes commonplace in neuropathic pain management.

When formulating a treatment plan for the patient with neuropathic pain there is no such thing as the 'best' option. Rather, a range of alternatives will exist that all have the potential for producing pain relief, but none of which will offer a therapeutic guarantee. Some patients will elect to try the simple topical preparations first. Usually they lack the potential for serious adverse effects and yet not infrequently produce pain relief. At the other end of the spectrum, acute and serious flare-ups of pain require immediately-acting agents. The existence of parenteral lidocaine, fosphenytoin, and 5HT$_3$ antagonists may remove the need to utilize immediate-release opioids with all their attendant side-effects.

Table 10.1 Dosing regimens for local anaesthetics and other co-analgesics

Drug	Dose	Dose interval	Time to effect
Topical			
Lidocaine	5% patch	one patch daily	days
Capsaicin	0.075%	four times daily	2–4 weeks
Doxepin	5% cream	four times daily	2 weeks
Oral			
Baclofen	10–20mg	three times daily	days
Tizanadine	4–8mg	three times daily	days
Mexiletine	50–150mg	four times daily	days
Ondansetron	4mg	three times daily	hours
Parenteral			
Lidocaine IV	500–1000mg	over 24 hours	immediate to 1 week
Phenytoin IV	600mg	over 24 hours	hours
Fosphenytoin IM	500PE*	once only	hours
Fosphenytoin IV	1000PE*	over 24 hours	hours
Ondansetron IV	8mg	once only	hours

*PE = 'phenytoin equivalent' units, the dose measure for fosphenytoin: 1 PE = 1mg phenytoin.

IV = intravenous, IM = intramuscular.

Cholecystokinin antagonists and cannabinoids not covered as currently commercially unavailable in UK.

Key references

Campbell, F.A., Tramer, M.R., Carroll, D., Reynolds, D.J., Moore, R.A., and McQuay, H.J. (2001). Are cannabinoids an effective and safe treatment option in the management of pain? A qualitative systematic review. *Br. Med. J.*; **323**, 1–6.

Mao, J. and Chen, L.L. (2000). Systemic lidocaine for neuropathic pain relief. *Pain*, **87**, 7–17.

McCleane, G.J. (2004). Cholecystokinin antagonists: a new way to improve analgesia from old analgesics? *Curr. Pharm. Des.*, **10**, 303–14.

McCleane, G.J. (2004). Pharmacological strategies in relieving neuropathic pain. *Expert Opin. Pharmacother.*, **5**, 1299–312.

Sawynok, J. (2003). Topically and peripherally acting analgesics. *Pharmacol. Rev.*, **55**, 1–20.

Chapter 11

Ketamine and other NMDA receptor antagonists

Marie T. Fallon and Cameron Fergus

Key points

- Ketamine is a non-competitive *N*-methyl D-aspartate (NMDA) receptor antagonist and is most effective in pain states where hyperexcitability is established.
- Ketamine undergoes first-pass metabolism to norketamine, which is a more potent analgesic than ketamine. This can explain why oral ketamine is more potent than parenteral ketamine.
- There is much clinical experience supporting use of ketamine in neuropathic pain states but the evidence base is not well established.
- Dextromethorphan is an alternative NMDA receptor antagonist and has been combined with morphine in some successful clinical trials.
- It is likely that more selective NMDA receptor subtype antagonists will be identified and developed in the future.

11.1 Ketamine pharmacology

11.1.1 Background

Ketamine is a dissociative anaesthetic agent which was developed in the 1960s. More recently, it has been used extensively in sub-anaesthetic doses for neuropathic pain of multiple aetiologies as well as for complex and refractory cancer pain, often in addition to opioids. Although there are relatively few randomized controlled trials of its use, there is a growing body of case report evidence for its effectiveness in the management of both cancer and non-cancer neuropathic pain.

11.1.2 **Pharmacodynamics**

The mode of action of ketamine is through non-competitive antagonism of the *N*-methyl D-aspartate (NMDA) receptor ion channel in the spinal cord (see Chapter 2). This channel, which is blocked by magnesium at rest, opens after excitation, a process involved in the development of opioid tolerance and wind-up. Ketamine interacts with the NMDA receptor phencyclidine binding site, significantly inhibiting the receptor activity – this occurs only after the channel has been opened (see Fig. 2.2., Chapter 2).

The effectiveness of ketamine is partially due to a wind-down phenomenon at the NMDA receptor, resetting the pain transmission pathway. In other words, it is most effective in pain states where hyperexcitability is established. Ketamine also interacts with opioid and muscarinic receptors, sodium and potassium channels, and inhibits serotonin and dopamine reuptake. This activity at multiple receptors means that ketamine can have unpleasant psychomimetic side-effects, including confusion, dysphoria, vivid dreams, and hallucinations. Other side-effects include hypertension and tachycardia. About 40% of patients will experience side-effects when ketamine is given by continuous subcutaneous infusion.

11.1.3 **Pharmacokinetics**

Ketamine undergoes first-pass metabolism to norketamine, which has lower *anaesthetic* potency than ketamine but probably has greater *analgesic* potency. Norketamine concentration is therefore greater after oral administration than parenteral administration, and norketamine may be responsible for most of the analgesic properties of ketamine. Norketamine is excreted renally.

11.1.4 **Preparations**

Standard ketamine exists as a racemic mixture of two stereoisomers: R (–) and S (+). S (+)-ketamine is now available and is more potent than R (–)-ketamine with fewer psychomimetic side-effects. Ketamine is usually given parenterally, most often intravenously or subcutaneously for chronic pain, or orally. It can also be given by the spinal or rectal route. There are reports of its use topically, as 0.5% ketamine cream, and intranasally as a spray.

11.2 **Clinical uses of ketamine**

11.2.1 **Peripheral neuropathic pain**

Controlled trials have demonstrated effective analgesia following intravenous (IV) ketamine for post-herpetic neuralgia and neuropathic pain following peripheral nerve injury due to surgery or chemotherapy. Although these trials have reported reduced allodynia and hyperalgesia, there was no effect on thermal sensitivity.

Continuous subcutaneous infusions of ketamine have been shown to relieve continuous pain in direct relationship to the dose of ketamine and the serum levels of ketamine and norketamine. However, side-effects, including induration at the site of infusion and psychomimetic reactions, were common. Despite this, patients often chose to continue the infusion, preferring the improved analgesia at the expense of side-effects. It is a useful adjuvant when other neuropathic agents have been unhelpful.

11.2.2 Central neuropathic pain

Ketamine has been described as reducing pain in patients with central dysaesthetic pain after spinal cord injury, following cauda equina trauma, and in central post-stroke pain after subarachnoid haemorrhage. In the latter case, a patient who described a constant, burning, generalized right-sided body pain with allodynia and hyperalgesia was treated successfully with ketamine after unsuccessful trials of epidural steroids, anti-epileptic, IV lidocaine, opioids, and antidepressants amongst others. She was titrated to 50mg three times a day of oral ketamine after a trial of IV ketamine and continued to have good analgesia after nine months without evidence of tolerance. Case histories such as this support the use of ketamine for pain where there are clinical features of central wind-up and which is not opioid responsive, or where the dose of opioid has to be limited because of side-effects.

11.2.3 Fibromyalgia

Two randomized controlled trials have shown non-significant benefit when comparing ketamine to morphine, lidocaine, naloxone, and placebo. It was suggested that the mechanism of action involved a reduction in central sensitization by ketamine.

11.2.4 Ischaemic pain

Ischaemic rest pain secondary to arteriosclerosis is thought to have both nociceptive and neuropathic elements and may be only partially opioid responsive. A double-blind randomized controlled trial compared regular opioids plus placebo, with regular opioids plus ketamine. This demonstrated statistically significant improvement in pain relief, general activity, and enjoyment of life, sustained up to five days after a single infusion.

11.2.5 Cancer pain

Unfortunately, there is a dearth of good-quality randomized controlled trials of ketamine in cancer pain. Four were identified as part of a recent Cochrane review but two of these were excluded because of inappropriate study design. The two accepted trials concluded that ketamine improves the effectiveness of morphine in the treatment of cancer pain. One trial compared ketamine 0.25mg/kg and 0.5mg/kg IV bolus with placebo in 10 cancer patients with neuropathic pain which was unrelieved by morphine. Ketamine significantly reduced the pain intensity in almost all the patients at both doses, with the effect being more marked at the higher dose. However, six out of 10 patients reported psychomimetic side-effects which were treated with diazepam.

The second accepted trial compared intrathecal morphine alone with intrathecal morphine plus ketamine in 20 patients with cancer neuropathic pain. The study suggested that ketamine enhanced the analgesic effect of morphine. No serious side-effects were reported in this study.

The Cochrane review concluded that there is insufficient data to enable any evidence-based conclusions about the benefits and harms of adjuvant ketamine alongside opioid therapy. However, there are many case reports and open-label trials describing the use of ketamine in combination with opioids. Many of these reports describe dramatic relief of pain in patients with refractory cancer pain. In most cases, the ketamine was used in addition to opioids, with treatment duration of between four hours and one year. Doses ranged from 1mg/kg/day by subcutaneous infusion to 600mg/day intravenously. Side-effects, including sedation and hallucinations, were generally not reported as severe.

11.2.6 Ketamine in children

Ketamine has been used as a pre-medication for painful procedures such as bone marrow aspiration and lumbar puncture in children. It has been reported as giving good analgesia with faster recovery time and fewer side-effects than alternatives.

There are individual case reports of ketamine used as an adjuvant to morphine in paediatric patients with cancer pain. One patient was a 12-year-old girl with severe neuropathic pain caused by a cervical spinal tumour which was not relieved by morphine. She was treated at home with IV ketamine for 67 days until her death. It is reported that she remained awake until the day before her death.

Another report discusses a two-year-old girl with severe pain from a metastatic neuroblastoma who was treated successfully with IV ketamine after an unsuccessful trial of methadone. The methadone was reported to cause unacceptable side-effects, including respiratory depression and sedation. Pain control was reasonable with ketamine and she was felt to have a better quality of life, as she was able to continue to communicate and to engage in activities.

11.3 Practical considerations

11.3.1 Patient selection

Clinical experience with ketamine is extensive, principally within the palliative care community but also within chronic pain clinics.

However, research evidence in support of various practices is more limited. Clinicians familiar with ketamine usually suggest that it is used for neuropathic pain that has not responded to standard approaches such as tricyclic antidepressants and anti-epileptics. It also has a place in cancer pain which is poorly or not responsive to opioids. Chronic pain states with features of central wind-up (allodynia, hyperalgesia, hyperpathia) in combination with poor opioid responsiveness will usually trigger a trial of ketamine.

Ketamine is contraindicated in patients with raised intracranial pressure, uncontrolled hypertension, psychosis, and epilepsy. It should be used with caution in patients with a history of cardiac failure or cerebrovascular disease. It may affect the hepatic metabolism of theophylline and levothyroxine.

Monitoring of blood pressure and pulse is recommended when starting or increasing ketamine (Table 11.1).

11.3.2 **Oral dosing**

An oral starting dose of 10mg four times daily is suggested, increased in 5–10mg increments daily until response is achieved. The usual oral dose range is 10–60mg four times daily, although there are reports of higher doses (up to 100mg qds) being used (Table 11.2). The parenteral formulation (10mg/ml) can be used but is extremely bitter – the taste can be masked with juice. There is now an oral preparation (50mg/5ml) available in the UK. This can be obtained by special order from Martindale Pharmaceuticals Ltd (see Appendix 1).

11.3.3 **Parenteral administration**

Ketamine is often administered by continuous subcutaneous infusion. The optimum dose is not clear but it is suggested that it is commenced at a low dose, e.g. 50–150mg/24 hours, by continuous subcutaneous infusion and increased in increments of 50–100mg daily (Table 11.2). Some specialists advise a reduction of regular opioid

Table 11.1 Ketamine in practice	
Contraindications	**Clinical management**
Uncontrolled hypertension Raised intracranial pressure Psychosis Epilepsy	
Cautions Cardiac failure Cerebrovascular disease	Monitor blood pressure and pulse
Adverse effects Psychomimetic (confusion, hallucinations, dysphoria)	Reduce dose, consider haloperidol or benzodiazepine

Table 11.2 **Ketamine dosing schedules**			
Route	Starting doses	Increments	Usual dose range
Oral (50mg/ml solution)	10mg qds	5–10mg per dose (20–40mg daily)	10–100mg qds
Subcutaneous infusion			
• Continuous	50–150mg/day	50–100mg daily	50–600mg/day
• Burst	50–150mg/day	100mg daily	100–500mg/day between 3 and 5 days only

dose by 33–50% at the start of ketamine treatment, or a switch to a short-acting opioid. The usual dose range is 50–600mg/day but doses of up to 2400mg/day have been reported.

Ketamine should be diluted with 0.9% saline and prepared daily. The addition of 1mg dexamethasone to the syringe driver and daily rotation of the site may prevent subcutaneous inflammation. Concomitant use of haloperidol or a benzodiazepine may be necessary to reduce the risk of psychomimetic side-effects. Once pain has stabilized with ketamine it may be continued for some time. There are reports of its use subcutaneously for over one year.

11.3.4 **Conversion from parenteral to oral dosing**

In some units, ketamine is started by the subcutaneous route in order to assess response. If there is a good response, conversion to the oral route may be attempted. Because of the first-pass metabolism from ketamine to its more potent active metabolite norketamine, oral ketamine is more potent than parenteral ketamine. The starting oral dose is not, therefore, related to the subcutaneous dose. Because of this, some clinicians now start treatment with oral ketamine and avoid the initial subcutaneous titration for those patients able to use the oral route. There are case reports of conversion from subcutaneous to oral ketamine (precipitated by a shortage of the parenteral formulation), where good analgesia was achieved with oral ketamine at doses of 30–40% of the previous parenteral dose.

11.3.5 **Burst ketamine**

Recently, ketamine has been used as a continuous subcutaneous infusion over a short duration (three to five days) at doses titrated between 100–500mg/24 hours – so-called 'burst ketamine'. Although there are no placebo-controlled trials of its use in this way, response rates of up to 67% have been reported to the initial infusion, with good maintenance of pain control for up to eight weeks after cessation of the ketamine.

11.4 Other NMDA receptor antagonists

11.4.1 Magnesium

As magnesium blocks the NMDA receptor ion channel at rest, there is interest in the use of magnesium in the treatment of neuropathic pain. There is some evidence that IV magnesium sulphate (30mg/kg over 30 minutes) may be effective as an analgesic in patients with post-herpetic neuralgia. Of particular note is that it appears to be safe and well tolerated.

Magnesium sulphate has also been used for the treatment of neuropathic pain due to brachial or lumbosacral plexus infiltration by cancer. Doses of 500mg and 1g were used with benefit and with minimal side-effects. The role of magnesium in the treatment of neuropathic pain should become clearer in the future, but it is not expected to have a large role in the therapeutic armamentarium.

11.4.2 Dextromethorphan

Dextromethorphan has been shown to have NMDA receptor antagonist activity in experimental settings. It was introduced in the 1950s as an alternative opioid to morphine. Its main use in the UK is as an antitussive. As such, it is an ingredient in low doses in many over-the-counter cough preparations. Clinical trials of its use for neuropathic pain have reported mixed results, although there is some evidence that it may potentiate the effect of opioids, resulting in equal analgesia at lower doses of morphine.

Morphidex™, a 1:1 combination of morphine and dextromethorphan, has been studied in the USA, with disappointing results overall. In those trials of Morphidex™ with positive results, equianalgesic effects were found at significantly lower morphine doses.

It has also been suggested that a good response to a small dose (0.1mg/kg) of IV ketamine is a useful predictor of the likelihood of response to oral dextromethorphan. Therefore, at present the role of dextromethorphan as an adjuvant treatment for neuropathic pain remains unclear. Although dextromethorphan (and perhaps magnesium) may have a role to play in the future management of neuropathic and difficult cancer pain, it is likely that more selective NMDA subtype antagonists will be identified and developed.

Key references

Bell, R., Eccleston, C., and Kalso, E. (2003). Ketamine as an adjuvant to opioids for cancer pain. *Cochrane Database of Systematic Reviews*, Issue 1. Art. No.: CD003351. DOI: 10.1002/14651858.CD003351.

Finlay, I. (1999). Ketamine and its role in cancer pain. *Pain Reviews,* **6**, 303–13.

Hocking, G. and Cousins, M.J. (2003). Ketamine in chronic pain management: an evidence-based review. *Anesth Analg.,* **97**, 1730–9.

Mitchell, A.C. and Fallon, M.T. (2002). A single infusion of intravenous ketamine improves pain relief in patients with critical limb ischaemia: results of a double blind randomised controlled trial. *Pain,* **97**, 275–81.

Chapter 12

Opioids

Michael I. Bennett

> **Key points**
>
> - Opioid receptor structure and function can be altered in neuropathic pain states, leading to reduced sensitivity to opioids.
> - Opioids were thought to be ineffective for neuropathic pain but substantial evidence exists to demonstrate analgesic efficacy, in some cases superior to more commonly used co-analgesics.
> - The most convincing evidence supports use of morphine, oxycodone, and tramadol in neuropathic pain.
> - Methadone, buprenorphine, and fentanyl may have a role but are supported by less convincing evidence, though the evidence base is growing rapidly.
> - Opioids should be used with caution in chronic pain management because of unknown long-term effects and risk of misuse. Adherence to local protocols and guidelines is recommended.

12.1 Opioids, opioid receptors, and neuropathic pain

12.1.1 History of opioids in neuropathic pain

The term 'opioid' includes naturally occurring, semi-synthetic, and synthetic drugs which, like morphine, combine with opioid receptors to produce their effects. An 'opiate' is a drug derived from the opium poppy, such as morphine and codeine.

The place of opioids in the management of neuropathic pain has been controversial until relatively recently. Clinical observations in the 1970s and 1980s of patients with nociceptive and neuropathic pain diagnoses who were given single doses of opioids suggested that neuropathic pain was resistant to opioids. These studies were often small, non-randomized, and uncontrolled, though their conclusions were readily taken up by some clinicians. By the 1990s, observational and controlled studies began to emerge that demonstrated dose responsiveness to opioids in patients with neuropathic pain. Although patients with nociceptive pain experienced greater pain relief, it was clear that neuropathic pain confers reduced sensitivity to opioids, rather than resistance. Over the last 10 years, much more consistent evidence has emerged to support the use of opioids as a class (as well as individual drugs) in the treatment of neuropathic pain.

12.1.2 Types of opioid receptors

There are at least three types of opioid receptor that mediate analgesia: μ (mu), κ (kappa), and δ (delta) (Table 12.1). A fourth receptor, called nociceptin orphanin FQ peptide (NOP), shares the structural characteristics of other opioid receptors but has low affinity for opioid agonists and antagonists. In clinical practice, therapeutic opioids are largely active at μ receptors and their effects are antagonized by naloxone. Recent research in animal models suggests that a novel form of the μ receptor may exist. This receptor binds diamorphine (heroin) and morphine-6-glucuronide (M6G) with high affinity, but has no interaction with morphine.

12.1.3 Opioid receptor activation

Opioid receptors are G-protein-coupled receptors and are found throughout the spinal cord and in many areas of the brain. Opioid receptors are located pre-synaptically on primary afferent neurons within the dorsal horn of the spinal cord. Once activated, they inhibit glutamate release and hence inhibit transmission of nociceptive stimuli from C and Aδ fibres.

Activated opioid receptors may also reduce gamma amino butyric acid (GABA) release within the peri-aquaductal grey (PAG), an area of the midbrain involved in the central control of nociceptive transmission. GABA is the main inhibitory transmitter in the brain and acts to reduce or prevent anti-nociceptive outflow descending to the spinal cord from the PAG. Thus the additional effect of opioids is to block GABA and therefore boost the descending inhibitory control pathway, reducing pain transmission.

Table 12.1 Opioid receptors	
Opioid receptor subtype	Effect of agonist
Mu	Analgesia, respiratory depression, reduced gastrointestinal motility, hypotension
Kappa	Analgesia, sedation, psychomimetic effects, some respiratory depression
Delta	Analgesia, respiratory depression
NOP	Little evidence of clinical effect of agonist or antagonist

12.1.4 Opioid receptors in neuropathic pain

Laboratory work has provided a number of explanations why neuropathic pain exhibits reduced sensitivity to opioids. This includes genetic variation in receptor sensitivity and in particular the influence of genetic polymorphisms. These are minor changes in the amino acid sequencing of receptors and their associated proteins that impact on opioid binding. Additional factors include loss of opioid receptors on pre-synaptic spinal terminals and up-regulation of the neuromodulator cholecystokinin (CCK) which antagonises opioid effects. Other evidence suggests that neuropathic pain causes opioid receptors themselves to become un-coupled from the G-proteins that they usually activate, resulting in lack of activity even if a drug binds to the opioid receptor.

12.1.5 Opioids and hypersensitivity

Emerging evidence suggests that the clinical effects of opioids are mediated not only by their analgesic or anti-nociceptive activity (the ability to reduce pain signals), but also by their ability to inhibit excitation or 'wind-up' processes (see also Chapter 2). Some opioids that are pure µ agonists are thought to induce excitation when used in large doses and there is some clinical evidence to support this. In contrast, opioids that have antagonist activity at certain receptors may inhibit processes that lead to excitation, e.g. methadone and buprenorphine. Evidence to support this is reviewed under each drug.

12.2 Morphine

12.2.1 Pharmacology

Morphine is a natural derivative of the opium poppy and is the prototypical µ receptor agonist. It is readily absorbed after oral administration, mainly in the upper small bowel, and is metabolized in the liver and at other sites to morphine-3-glucuronide (M3G) and M6G. M6G is an active metabolite and is a more potent analgesic than morphine. Morphine and its glucuronides are renally excreted and so may accumulate with impaired renal function.

Morphine is available as oral normal-release and sustained-release preparations, as well as injections. Normal-release oral preparations of morphine generally produce analgesic effects within one hour (oral solution is faster than tablets), with a plasma half-life of around two hours. Sustained-release preparations are effective within two to three hours, with a plasma half-life of approximately six to eight hours.

12.2.2 Clinical studies

Morphine was originally thought to improve mood alone, rather than pain, in patients with neuropathic pain. Single-dose and longer-term

Table 12.2 Opioid activity at receptor sites

	Mu	Kappa	Delta	NOP	NMDA	Serotonergic	Noradrenergic
Morphine	+						
Oxycodone	+	+					
Fentanyl	++						
Tramadol	+					+	+
Methadone	+				−		
Buprenorphine	(+)	−	−				
Diamorphine	+						

+ = full agonist
(+) = partial agonist
− = antagonist

studies in patients with post-herpetic neuralgia, however, showed that morphine is as effective as intravenous (IV) lidocaine and oral tricyclic antidepressants, and all these treatments were significantly better than placebo. A well-designed study compared morphine, gabapentin, placebo, and combined morphine/gabapentin in a group of patients with post-herpetic neuralgia or diabetic neuropathy. This showed that morphine produced as good pain relief as gabapentin in these patients (in fact, slightly better – see Chapter 16 for more details).

In central neuropathic pain, morphine has also been shown to reduce brush-evoked allodynia compared to placebo in the short term, but was less successful in the longer term, at one year.

12.3 **Oxycodone**

12.3.1 **Pharmacology**

Oxycodone is a semi-synthetic opioid with many similarities to morphine. A potentially important difference is that oxycodone has activity at both μ and κ opioid receptors. Activity at this additional site has been used to explain the effectiveness of oxycodone in neuropathic pain and a reduction in adverse cognitive effects compared to morphine (though possibly a higher incidence of constipation). Oxycodone has a high oral to parenteral availability and a twofold greater potency than morphine (i.e. 1mg oral oxycodone = 2mg oral morphine). It is metabolized to inactive substances.

Oxycodone is available as normal-release tablets and solution, and controlled-release preparations, as well as injections. In the USA oxycodone is available in combination with paracetamol and has proved a very useful drug for both cancer and non-cancer chronic pain. Parenteral preparations allow continuity of analgesic effect for patients treated with oral oxycodone who are no longer able to take oral medicine, for example peri-operatively or in a palliative care context.

12.3.2 **Clinical studies**

Clinical studies of controlled-release oxycodone have provided strong evidence of efficacy in the management of neuropathic pain. Two relatively small randomized controlled trials (RCTs) of less than 40 patients have been conducted in post-herpetic neuralgia and in diabetic neuropathy (though one used an active placebo to mimic side-effects). These studies showed significant improvements in the treatment arm compared to placebo, even though adverse effects were greater with treatment. Another larger RCT in diabetic neuropathy, conducted over six weeks, also showed a significant reduction in pain ratings compared to placebo.

In all these studies, ongoing and spontaneous pains were improved, and significant reductions in pain interference scores were noted, without changes in scores of mood. These data suggest that oxy-codone can improve neuropathic pain and functioning and that these improvements are not brought about by changes in mood. Meta-analyses show that the number needed to treat (NNT) for oxycodone is 2.5. This means that one in every 2.5 (or four out of 10) patients with neuropathic pain treated with this drug will get around 50% reduction in their pain.

12.4 **Fentanyl**

12.4.1 **Pharmacology**

Fentanyl is a very potent synthetic opioid that is quickly metabolized to the inactive metabolite norfentanyl and excreted via the kidneys. It is approximately 100 times as potent as morphine (1mg fentanyl = 100mg morphine) and is safe to use in patients with renal impairment or renal failure, in contrast to morphine.

Fentanyl is highly lipophilic, meaning that it is readily absorbed into tissue containing fat and is therefore ideal for topical use. Fentanyl is available as transdermal patches that deliver a steady release of fentanyl into a subcutaneous depot over a three-day period. However, fentanyl clearance is slower in elderly patients and so sustained-release prepara-tions should be used with caution in this population. It is also available as oral transmucosal fentanyl citrate lozenges for absorption onto the buccal mucosa. These can provide rapid release of fentanyl and are often used to control cancer breakthrough pain, though there is no evidence to support their specific use in neuropathic pain.

12.4.2 **Clinical studies**

Studies in the late 1990s showed that single-dose IV fentanyl provided significantly better relief of neuropathic pain, compared to either diaze-pam or placebo, in patients with a variety of neuropathic pain diagno-ses. Based on this success, the research group logically thought that continuation with fentanyl therapy, in the form of sustained-release transdermal patches, should be tested. In the open-label trial, the origi-nal patients did not do as well when followed up over a four-week period. Only a third felt some relief of their pain; the other two-thirds experienced no improvement or adverse effects leading to withdrawal.

12.5 **Tramadol**

12.5.1 **Pharmacology**

Tramadol is often considered a weak opioid in contrast to the strong opioids morphine, oxycodone, and fentanyl. It is active at μ opioid receptors as well as enhancing central serotonergic and noradrenergic inhibition of pain. Although these additional actions are thought to enhance its analgesic effects, they may also be responsible for additional antimuscarinic adverse effects. Tramadol is around five to eight times less potent than morphine (i.e. 50–80mg tramadol = 10mg morphine). Preparations are available as normal-release and sustained-release tablets.

12.5.2 **Clinical studies**

Tramadol has been evaluated in separate RCTs of patients with post-herpetic neuralgia and diabetic neuropathy. These studies have provided a reasonable evidence base for demonstrating its effectiveness in neuropathic pain. A Cochrane review found that the NNT for tramadol is 3.5, meaning that two patients in seven with neuropathic pain will get about 50% reduction in their pain with tramadol.

12.6 **Methadone**

12.6.1 **Pharmacology**

Methadone is a synthetic opioid and is well absorbed after oral administration. Its effects are largely mediated through μ opioid receptors but it exists as a racemic mixture. L-methadone produces opioid effects but D-methadone is active at NMDA receptors (see Chapters 2 and 11). Its average half-life is 24 hours, although this may vary between eight and 80 hours in different individuals, and there is a clear age-related increase in half-life. Methadone should be used with extreme caution, particularly in the elderly, because its unpredictable half-life means that accumulation may occur. This also means that its potency ratio to morphine has been difficult to establish. Best estimates suggest it is five to 10 times more potent than morphine with chronic administration (i.e. regular dosing with methadone 10mg = regular dosing with 50–100mg of morphine). It is metabolized to inactive substances.

12.6.2 **Clinical studies**

In neuropathic pain, methadone has been shown to have significantly better analgesic effects than placebo when given over a two-week period to patients with a mixture of neuropathic pain diagnoses. Whether methadone is superior to other opioids because of its NMDA receptor activity has yet to be demonstrated. Indeed, various studies have examined conversion ratios of morphine to methadone in patients with chronic pain. A higher ratio (signifying less methadone required for the same degree of pain relief, compared to morphine) was not seen in patients with neuropathic pain. This suggests that NMDA activity is minimal and that it is the μ agonist activity of methadone that results in the principal analgesic effect.

However, anecdotal reports exist describing the successful use of methadone in patients with severe cancer neuropathic pain previously treated with morphine. These patients had exhibited signs of excitation or hypersensitivity on large doses of morphine (generalized allodynia, myoclonus, increasing doses led to worse pain), but were well controlled on relatively low doses of methadone. Whether this success was due to NMDA antagonism or just a reduction in overall opioid dose is not clear.

12.7 **Buprenorphine**

12.7.1 **Pharmacology**

Buprenorphine is a partial μ agonist but has antagonist actions at κ and δ opioid receptors. It is available as sublingual tablets and more recently as transdermal patches that are similar in action to fentanyl patches. Buprenorphine is metabolized to inactive substances. Animal and volunteer studies suggest that buprenorphine has the highest antihyperalgesic effect of all opioids, i.e. it is most able to inhibit excitation.

12.7.2 **Clinical studies**

Clinical evidence supporting a role for buprenorphine in neuropathic pain is only just emerging and currently is not as strong as for some other opioids. Case series exist describing the effective use of buprenorphine in post-thoracotomy neuropathic pain and in cases where other opioids have failed to control pain dominated by neuropathic features. Further research is needed to examine whether the theoretical advantages of buprenorphine translate into clinical effectiveness.

12.8 **Diamorphine**

No specific evidence supports the use of diamorphine in neuropathic pain. This is probably because it is only available in a few countries, mainly the UK (and specifically not the USA where many drug studies are conducted), and has always been thought of as a pro-drug for morphine. The cloning of a novel μ receptor that is activated by diamorphine and M6G, and not morphine, may lead to new research on diamorphine in neuropathic pain.

Anecdotally (and in a palliative care setting), some patients with cancer neuropathic pain do experience greater analgesia with diamorphine via injection or subcutaneous infusion, than with oral morphine. This is often regarded as illogical or counter-intuitive, but could be explained by differences in opioid receptor expression and activity. Diamorphine is highly soluble and this allows large doses to be given in very small volumes.

12.9 **Opioids in clinical practice**

12.9.1 **Need for caution**

Although there is now a large body of evidence demonstrating the analgesic *efficacy* of opioids in neuropathic pain, a number of concerns exist about the *effectiveness* of opioids in clinical practice. These relate to well-described adverse effects that appear in the short term, fears about tolerance and addiction, and relatively unknown long-term, and potentially irreversible, effects of opioids. However, there is no doubt that opioids have a role in both cancer and non-cancer neuropathic pain. In the latter context, careful selection and adherence to local protocols, that may include patient contracts, may be necessary.

12.9.2 **Common adverse effects**

Common adverse effects that can appear relatively soon after initiating treatment with opioids include somnolence and other cognitive effects, nausea, and constipation (Table 12.3). Sedation is common when commencing morphine and after the dose has been increased. It usually wears off after two to three days at the same dose, and patients on stable doses of morphine can be allowed to drive. Hallucinations, confusion, and vivid dreams may necessitate a dose reduction or a change to an alternative opioid; alternatively they can be managed with a small dose of haloperidol (1.5–3mg) at night. Side-effects should be discussed with patients before they decide to commence opioids. There is no evidence that patients on chronic opioids are cognitively impaired or are unable to drive safely. However, patients must be warned about driving when commencing opioids. They should be advised not to drive for one to two weeks after commencing treatment or increasing dose and that their insurance company may need to be informed of all medication that they are taking.

All opioids can cause nausea (30–50% of patients), vomiting (10% of patients), and constipation (around 80%). Constipation is usually greatest when commencing opioids. There is some evidence to support the concept that tolerance may develop to the constipating effects of opioids over time, and that a ceiling effect of opioid-induced constipation is reached relatively early. In other words, once established on opioids, patients may not be any more constipated if the dose is increased. All patients commenced on opioids should be prescribed softening and stimulant laxatives and have access to an anti-emetic. Other well-recognized side-effects are dry mouth, itching, sweating, myoclonic jerks, and occasionally hypotension.

Respiratory depression is unusual but may occur in opioid-naive patients given a large dose of an opioid for acute pain, or due to a drug error or accumulation of opioid in the very elderly or its metabolites in renal failure. In chronic use, tolerance to the respiratory depressant effects occurs rapidly and provided the dose is titrated against the patient's pain, opioids can be used safely, even in patients with chronic lung disease. A physiological explanation for this is that the respiratory centre receives nociceptive input which counterbalances the respiratory potential of the opioid.

12.9.3 Fears about tolerance and addiction

Both professionals and patients have fears about the use of strong opioids, particularly morphine (Table 12.4). These fears are largely unfounded and with careful, knowledgeable use there are few problems. However, since these fears are common and may lead to poor pain management, the professional will need to discuss these issues with the patient when commencing strong opioids.

Tolerance is the need for a higher dose to achieve the same pharmacological effect. There is no doubt (from experimental studies in acute pain) that tolerance to opioids can occur, possibly through down-regulation of opioid receptors after prolonged exposure to opioid agonists. The clinically relevant issue is to what extent this can be managed by careful patient selection, opioid switching (see Chapter 16), or alternative combinations of analgesics.

Patients with cancer-related pain often have an unfounded fear that if they start taking opioids, the drugs won't work later, when they really need it. An increase in analgesic requirement is usually due to an increase in pain due to advancing disease, rather than to tolerance.

Table 12.3 Opioid side-effects

Side-effect	Generally dose related?	Management strategy
Dry mouth	No	Frequent mouth care, artificial saliva
Constipation	Probably not	Prophylactic laxative, e.g. co-danthramer
Nausea	Yes	Tends to wear off, regular metoclopramide if not
Sedation or confusion	Yes	Reduce dose by 30%, check renal function, may respond to change of opioid
Hallucinations	Yes	Reduce dose by 30%, consider haloperidol, may respond to change of opioid
Pruritus	No	May respond to change of opioid

Table 12.4 Fears about opioid use	
Professional's fears	Patient's fears
Addiction	Addiction
Respiratory depression	Side-effects
Excess sedation	Tolerance
Confusion	Decreased options for future pain relief

Addiction does not occur when opioids are used carefully for the management of pain. If the cause of the pain is removed (e.g. by a nerve block or healing of an injury) then opioids can generally be reduced or withdrawn with no psychological problems. Occasionally there is a degree of *physical* dependence, with a physical withdrawal syndrome apparent upon withdrawal of the drug. This is characterized by fatigue, yawning, lacrimation, myalgia/arthralgia, and anxiety through to tachycardia, abdominal cramps, diarrhoea, nausea, and insomnia in more severe cases. However, when the opioid is withdrawn in staged decrements, this is easily managed.

Psychological dependence is a compulsion to continue to take the opioid because of the need for stimulation or because it relieves anxiety. Only a very small proportion of patients with chronic pain will develop psychological dependence. If there is drug-seeking behaviour or the apparent rapid development of tolerance to opioids in an otherwise stable pain (exclude disease progression or deterioration), clinicians should urgently review the patient and this may require the help of a specialist addiction service. Helpful guidelines on the use of opioids in patients with chronic non-cancer-related pain can be found on the British Pain Society's website (see Appendix 1).

12.9.4 Long-term effects of opioids

Many studies of opioids in chronic neuropathic pain are of relatively short duration – days to weeks. In clinical practice, commencing a patient on opioids may result in months or years of treatment and the long-term effects of opioids are relatively unknown. Current concerns relate to the long-term opioid effects on endocrine and immune systems. Specifically, infertility and suppressed immunity are potential consequences. Babies born of women who take long-term opioids may develop respiratory depression at birth and require specialist help.

Key references

Boureau, F., Legallicier, P., and Marmar, K. (2003). Tramadol in postherpetic neuralgia: a randomized, double-blind, placebo-controlled trial. *Pain*, **104**, 323–31.

Dellemijn, P.L., van Duijn, H., and Vanneste, J.A. (1998). Prolonged treatment with transdermal fentanyl in neuropathic pain. *J. Pain Symptom Manage.*, **16**, 220–9.

Gilron, I., Bailey, J.M., Dongsheng, T., Holden, R.R., Weaver, D.F., and Houlden, R.L. (2005). Morphine, gabapentin, or their combination for neuropathic pain. *N. Engl. J. Med.*, **352**, 1324–34.

Koppert, W., Ihmsen, H., Korber, N., Wehrfritz, A., Sittl, R., Schmelz, M., et al. (2005). Different profiles of buprenorphine-induced analgesia and antihyperalgesia in a human pain model. *Pain*, **118**, 15–22.

Morley, J.S., Bridson, J., Nash, T., Miles, J.B., White, S., and Makin, M.K. (2003). Low-dose methadone has an analgesic effect in neuropathic pain: a double-blind randomised controlled crossover trial. *Palliat. Med.*, **17**, 576–87.

Simonnet, G. (2005). Opioids: from analgesia to antihyperalgesia? *Pain*, **118**, 8–9.

Watson, C.P., Moulin, D., Watt-Watson, J., Gordon, A., and Eisenhoffer, J. (2003). Controlled-release oxycodone relieves neuropathic pain: a randomized controlled trial in painful diabetic neuropathy. *Pain*, **105**, 71–8.

Chapter 13

Transcutaneous electrical nerve stimulation (TENS) and acupuncture

Mark I. Johnson

Key points

- TENS and acupuncture are simple and generally safe methods of stimulating peripheral nerves and muscles close to the site of pain in order to modulate nociceptive input to the spinal cord.
- TENS can be useful for peripheral neuropathic pain and analgesic effects are often felt immediately.
- Best results occur when patients are given a supervised trial of TENS to guide electrode placement and stimulation settings, although TENS is widely available to the public.
- Pain relief from acupuncture is generally delayed following treatment but often outlasts the stimulation period (in contrast to TENS).
- There is a dearth of good-quality evidence to guide decisions regarding TENS and acupuncture in neuropathic pain. However, both have few adverse effects, can be combined easily with drug therapy, and are always worth a trial in a patient who has not responded to other treatments.

13.1 Transcutaneous electrical nerve stimulation (TENS)

13.1.1. Background

Transcutaneous electrical nerve stimulation (TENS) is the delivery of pulsed electrical currents across the intact surface of the skin to stimulate the underlying nerves. A battery-powered, portable stimulating device is used to generate the currents, and conducting pads called electrodes are used to deliver the currents through the skin (Fig. 13.1).

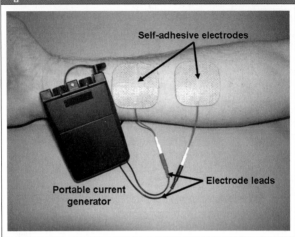

Fig 13.1 Standard TENS device

Self-adhesive electrodes

Electrode leads

Portable current generator

TENS is non-invasive, easy to administer, and has few side-effects or drug interactions. TENS effects are immediate for most patients and there is no potential for toxicity or overdose. TENS treatment is cheap when compared to long-term drug therapy. At the time of writing, a standard TENS device costs approximately £30 (approx. €43) and running costs (batteries and electrodes) are low. Patients can administer TENS themselves at home and titrate the dosage of treatment as required. Patients can purchase TENS devices over the counter without medical prescription, although new patients should always be given a supervised trial of TENS from a practitioner experienced in the principles of application. Patients should be provided with a point of contact to troubleshoot any problems with TENS.

13.1.2 Biological rationale and plausibility

The physiological purpose of TENS is to selectively activate large-diameter non-noxious afferents (Aβ) without activating smaller-diameter nociceptive afferents (Aδ and C). Physiological studies have shown that Aβ afferent input inhibits ongoing activity in second-order nociceptive neurons in the dorsal horn of the spinal cord.

13.1.3 Clinical effectiveness

Clinical experience suggests that TENS is useful for neuropathic pain, irrespective of cause and whether or not there is a sympathetic component. TENS appears to be more effective for neuropathic pains of peripheral rather than central origin, especially if there is a loss of large-fibre input. However, there are few good-quality randomized controlled clinical trials.

Published trials suggest that TENS is beneficial for peripheral neuropathic pain due to post-herpetic neuralgia, trigeminal neuralgia, phantom limb and stump pain, radiculopathies (cervical, thoracic, and lumbar), diabetes, and entrapment neuropathies such as carpal tunnel syndrome. TENS has been used for neuropathic cancer pain caused by nerve compression by a neoplasm or infiltration by a tumor, and for iatrogenic neuralgias such as post-mastectomy and post-thoracotomy pains. TENS may also be useful for complex regional pain syndromes type I (reflex sympathetic dystrophy) and type II (causalgia), and central pain states following stroke and post-traumatic spinal cord injury pain. A Cochrane review on electrical stimulation for post-stroke pain was inconclusive.

13.2 TENS: principles of use

13.2.1 Electrode position

TENS electrodes must be positioned on healthy skin where sensation is intact, so it is important to check skin sensation prior to application. TENS may aggravate neuropathic pain, especially when there is mechanical (tactile) allodynia. Therefore, electrodes should be positioned along the main nerves well proximal to the site of pain in the first instance. Alternatively, electrodes can be positioned on a contralateral dermatome or paravertebrally at the appropriate spinal segment. For most other types of pain, TENS electrodes are placed around the site of pain so that paraesthesia can be directed into the painful area (Fig. 13.2a and b).

13.2.2 Electrical characteristics of TENS

The potential number of TENS protocols is vast (Fig. 13.3). Theoretically, selective activation of large-diameter afferents occurs best with high-frequency (e.g. 10–200 pulses per second), low-intensity currents with pulse durations between 50–500µs. In practice, activation of large-diameter afferents is recognized by a 'strong but comfortable' paraesthesia beneath the electrodes and patients are instructed to titrate the intensity of currents to achieve this effect. Patients are encouraged to experiment with TENS settings for pulse frequency, pulse pattern, and pulse duration because optimal settings remain unknown.

13.2.3 Timing and dosage

TENS effects are often immediate and are maximal when the device is switched on. Hence, patients should keep the device switched on whenever they need pain relief. Patients can leave electrodes *in situ* and administer TENS intermittently throughout the day, providing

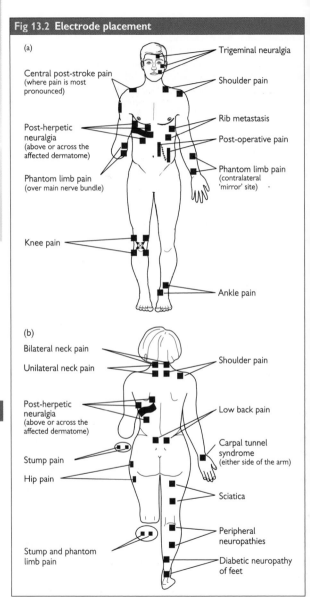

Fig 13.2 Electrode placement

(a)

Trigeminal neuralgia

Central post-stroke pain (where pain is most pronounced)

Shoulder pain

Rib metastasis

Post-herpetic neuralgia (above or across the affected dermatome)

Post-operative pain

Phantom limb pain (over main nerve bundle)

Phantom limb pain (contralateral 'mirror' site)

Knee pain

Ankle pain

(b)

Bilateral neck pain

Unilateral neck pain

Shoulder pain

Post-herpetic neuralgia (above or across the affected dermatome)

Low back pain

Carpal tunnel syndrome (either side of the arm)

Stump pain

Hip pain

Sciatica

Peripheral neuropathies

Stump and phantom limb pain

Diabetic neuropathy of feet

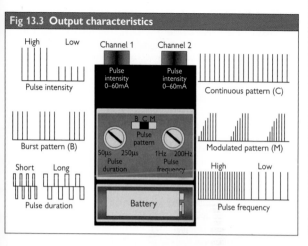

Fig 13.3 Output characteristics

High — Low
Pulse intensity

Burst pattern (B)

Short — Long
Pulse duration

Channel 1   Channel 2

Pulse intensity 0–60mA   Pulse intensity 0–60mA

B C M
Pulse pattern

50µs   250µs
Pulse duration

1Hz   200Hz
Pulse frequency

Battery

Continuous pattern (C)

Modulated pattern (M)

High — Low
Pulse frequency

they attend to skin care underneath the electrodes as minor skin irritation may occur. Patients should wash skin after TENS and should apply electrodes to adjacent fresh skin on a regular basis.

13.2.4 Contraindications and precautions

Patients with cardiac pacemakers or with cardiac problems should not use TENS, unless the situation has been discussed with their cardiologist. TENS should not be administered over the abdomen or pelvis during pregnancy because its effects on fetal development are unknown and currents could inadvertently cause uterine contractions. Practitioners should be cautious when giving TENS to patients with epilepsy as it may be difficult to exclude it as a potential cause of a seizure. TENS should not be given to patients with a history of autonomic reactions to tactile allodynia such as syncope, or to patients with compromised circulation such as thrombosis. Decisions are left to the discretion of the medical practitioner.

TENS should not be applied internally (mouth), over areas of broken or damaged skin, or over the anterior part of the neck as this may cause an acute hypotensive response. TENS should not be used while operating motor vehicles or potentially hazardous equipment or while in the shower or bath. It can be used at bedtime providing the device has a timer so that it automatically switches off. It can also be used on children providing they understand what to expect during the process.

13.2.5 Acupuncture-like TENS (AL-TENS)

This technique can be used when patients do not respond to conventional TENS. Electrodes are placed over motor points at myotomes related to the origin of the pain and non-painful phasic

121

muscle contractions are generated using intermittent bursts of pulses generated by the TENS device (Fig. 13.3). The resultant input from small-diameter muscle afferents (ergoreceptors) activates descending inhibitory pain pathways which produces pain relief that outlasts the stimulation period. AL-TENS is given intermittently throughout the day, e.g. 20 minutes, three times a day.

Clinical experience suggests that AL-TENS is useful for radiating neuropathic pain such as sciatica and cervical rhizopathy. A dual-channel device (four electrodes) can be used to deliver conventional TENS over the nerve root as it emerges from the spinal cord and AL-TENS over the main muscle mass of the radiating pain. AL-TENS can be applied to contralateral myotomes when it is not possible to achieve TENS paraesthesia at the site of pain due to hyperaesthesia, hypoaesthesia, or dysaesthesia.

A variety of TENS-like devices are available on the market but their use is limited because of a lack of research evidence. They include microcurrent stimulation, transcutaneous spinal electroanalgesia (TSE), interferential therapy (IFT), and Pain® Gone pens.

13.3 **Acupuncture**

13.3.1 **Background**

Acupuncture is the technique of inserting fine needles through the skin into selected points in the body to stimulate underlying nerve and muscle tissue. Additional stimulation is achieved by 'twirling' the inserted needle or by passing mild currents through pairs of needles using a portable electrical stimulator, termed 'electroacupuncture'.

Originally, acupuncture was based on the principles of traditional Chinese medicine where it was believed that acupuncture could alter the flow of vital energies of life (Yin and Yang) along energy channels or meridians. Nowadays, many medical practitioners adopt a Western approach to acupuncture which involves diagnosis according to orthodox medicine.

13.3.2 **Biological rationale and plausibility**

There is no convincing evidence for the existence of meridians as finite structures. Evidence that acupuncture points correspond to anatomical structures such as nerve bundles, nerves emerging from deep to superficial motor points, myofascial trigger points, and perivascular plexi has been challenged.

Needling during acupuncture stimulates high-threshold receptors and/or their afferents (Aδ and C), leading to segmental and extrasegmental modulation of nociceptive input. Post-stimulation effects have been attributed to activity in descending inhibitory pain pathways, the release of endogenous opioids, and positive-feedback neural circuitry in the mesolimbic region of the brain.

Acupuncture affects activity in the autonomic nervous system and may improve microcirculation through axon reflexes and the release of vasoactive substances such as calcitonin gene-related peptide and substance P.

13.3.3 Clinical effectiveness

Clinical experience suggests that acupuncture is beneficial for nociceptive and musculoskeletal pain but is less effective for neuropathic pain. Beneficial effects have been reported on phantom limb pain, diabetic neuropathy, and neurogenic pruritus. A randomized, placebo-controlled, multicentre clinical trial found that acupuncture was no more effective than placebo for peripheral neuropathy in human immunodeficiency virus (HIV) infected individuals. A recent systematic review concluded that rigorous clinical trials do not support acupuncture as an effective analgesic adjunctive method for pain related to cancer, including neuropathic pain. However, there are insufficient good-quality randomized controlled trials to guide clinical decisions for neuropathic pain conditions. For this reason, acupuncture may be worth a trial in a patient who has not responded to other treatments or who cannot tolerate drug therapy. Acupuncture has few adverse effects and can be combined with drug therapy or TENS.

13.4 Acupuncture: principles of use

13.4.1 Point selection

Formal training is required to administer acupuncture (www.medical-acupuncture.co.uk). The exact site and depth of penetration is determined by the practitioner and believed to be critical to outcome. Western practitioners choose points in accordance with known physiological and anatomical principles, e.g. dermatome, myotome, and sclerotome. The general consensus is to use points from innervated regions with properly functioning nerves. Direct stimulation of hyperaesthetic areas is avoided.

Needles should be placed proximal to the site of nerve damage or above a complete transection in spinal cord injuries. Needles could be placed to surround a stump scar for phantom limb pain or on trigger areas in the stump, providing they are not hyperaesthetic. In conditions like post-herpetic neuralgia or trigeminal neuralgia, practitioners would stimulate above and below the affected segment or use contralateral 'mirror' points.

Points are avoided in areas of skin where the nerve supply or circulation has been compromised, as in peripheral neuropathy. Stronger stimulation acupuncture techniques such as electroacupuncture are often used if distant points are chosen. Trigger points are often used for pains of musculoskeletal origin. In practice, optimal point selection is achieved through a careful process of trial and error.

13.4.2 Timing and dosage

Acupuncturists typically use fine (0.2–0.3mm) disposable steel needles which are 30mm long. Needles are left in place for up to 30 minutes and may be intermittently manipulated to facilitate stimulation. Patients may report sensations of heaviness, soreness, a local dull ache, referred pain, numbness, and/or paraesthesia during acupuncture.

In general, pain relief from acupuncture outlasts the period of stimulation and may persist for several days or weeks. The onset of analgesia may be delayed and some patients experience an initial transient increase in pain in the first 48 hours. A typical course of acupuncture consists of six to 12 treatments given once per week. Pain relief may be cumulative over time. Patients may attend acupuncture clinics for 'top-up' sessions thereafter.

13.4.3 Contraindications and precautions

Acupuncture is relatively safe when administered by a trained practitioner. Contraindications include bleeding disorders, anticoagulant medication, placing needles close to a pregnant uterus, and patients with a needle phobia.

Electroacupuncture is contraindicated for patients with cardiac pacemakers. Serious adverse events such as pneumothorax, cardiac tamponade, and fatalities due to needle infection are rare, although minor events such as pain due to the needles, tiredness, and bleeding are much more common. Occasionally patients may feel faint.

Key references

Barlas, P. and Lundeberg, T. (2006). Transcutaneous electrical nerve stimulation and acupuncture. In: S.B. McMahaon and M. Koltzenburg (ed.) *Melzack and Wall's textbook of pain*, pp. 583–90. Elsevier Churchill Livingstone, Philadelphia.

Johnson, M.I. (2002). Transcutaneous electrical nerve stimulation. In: S.M. Kitchen (ed.) *Electrotherapy: evidence-based practice*, pp.259–86, Churchill Livingstone, Edinburgh, UK.

Lee, H., Schmidt, K., and Ernst, E. (2005). Acupuncture for the relief of cancer-related pain: a systematic review. *Eur. J. Pain*, **9**: 437–44.

National Health Service Centre for Reviews and Dissemination (2001). Acupuncture. *Effective Health Care Bulletin*, **7**: 1–2

Price, C.I. and Pandyan, A.D. (2001). Electrical stimulation for preventing and treating post-stroke shoulder pain: a systematic Cochrane review. *Clin. Rehab.*, **15**: 5–19.

Shlay, J.C., Chaloner, K., Max, M.B., Flaws, B., Reichelderfer, P., Wentworth, D., *et al.* (1998). Acupuncture and amitriptyline for pain due to HIV-related peripheral neuropathy: a randomized controlled trial. *J.A.M.A.* **280**: 1590–5.

Chapter 14

Spinal cord stimulation

Brian A. Simpson

> ## Key points
>
> - Electricity has been used for centuries to relieve pain but spinal cord stimulation (SCS) came about with the Gate Control Theory in the 1960s.
> - SCS was originally thought simply to 'close the gate' by activating Aβ fibres but its effect is more complex. It is likely that it helps to normalize the dysfunction that manifests as neuropathic pain.
> - SCS is most effective for ischaemic and neuropathic pain, and is ineffective in nociceptive pain.
> - Electrodes are placed in the epidural space either via percutaneous needle or at open operation. The power source is usually implanted and is similar to a cardiac pacemaker.
> - SCS can produce significant benefits in terms of pain and function in up to 70% of patients with neuropathic pain, though more controlled trials are needed to establish long-term benefits.

14.1 Introduction

14.1.1 Electricity and pain relief

There is nothing new about the use of electricity to relieve pain. Natural sources, particularly electric fish and also the static electricity from amber, etc., were widely used for thousands of years. Man-made electricity dates from 1672 (electrostatic generator) and could be stored after 1745 (Leyden jar). Electroacupuncture is nearly 200 years old (1823) and peripheral nerve stimulation was also developed during the nineteenth century. It was very widely employed but its widespread misuse led to its ban in the USA in 1910. History nearly repeated itself in the 1970s and early 1980s with spinal cord stimulation (SCS).

14.1.2 **Modern neurostimulation**

The modern era of therapeutic neurostimulation was triggered in the 1960s by the gate theory of pain. It was the underlying principle, combined with a new appreciation of the plasticity of the nervous system and its tendency to generate pain when damaged, that fostered this modulatory approach along with a slow rejection of neurodestructive procedures. However, the combination of unreliable equipment, a lack of appreciation of the indications, and large numbers of practitioners each performing small numbers of procedures with inadequate follow-up almost led to its demise. Through improvements in each of these areas therapeutic neurostimulation not only survived but is developing rapidly, with many thousands of devices, mainly spinal cord stimulators, implanted annually worldwide. Despite the maturity and the breadth of the field, there are still fundamental issues to be resolved.

14.2 **Mechanism of action**

14.2.1 **Analgesic effects**

A great deal is still not known about how SCS works. The posterior columns have a key role and SCS is still sometimes referred to as 'dorsal column stimulation'. The large, myelinated, low-threshold Aβ afferent fibres, whose activity was proposed to 'close the gate' by inhibiting simultaneous nociceptive activity in small, unmyelinated C fibres, have collateral branches which ascend in the posterior columns. The rationale of SCS originally was to activate these Aβ collaterals, which transmit signals from mechanoreceptors: the electrophysiological equivalent of 'rubbing it better'.

There is an essential topographic element in that the electrodes must not only be ipsilateral (for unilateral pain), but stimulation must also evoke paraesthesiae which cover the painful area. Although the debate about the relative contributions of a supraspinal long-loop mechanism and an action at segmental level in the spinal cord continues, it is obvious that SCS does not simply close the gate on nociceptive input; it is not effective against nociceptive pain.

In animal models of neuropathic pain, the suppression of allodynia and of neuronal hyperexcitability in the dorsal horn of the spinal cord by SCS has been linked to an increased release of gamma amino butyric acid (GABA) and a decreased release of excitatory amino acids. Adenosine is also involved and neuronal activity changes have been demonstrated in brainstem nuclei.

14.2.2 **Anti-ischaemic effect**

SCS has an anti-ischaemic effect and the extent to which this underlies the analgesic effect in ischaemic pain is not yet established. It also stabilizes the vasomotor and sudomotor abnormalities in complex regional pain syndrome (CRPS) to a variable extent and appears to be able to reduce gastrointestinal spasm. There is as yet no consensus as to whether the autonomic effects represent modulation of ongoing sympathetic efferent activity or an antidromic activation of primary afferents.

Neuropathic pain is the product of a complex dysfunction of the nervous system and it seems that SCS produces a degree of normalization, probably by several mechanisms whose relative contribution varies in different conditions.

14.3 Selection of cases

14.3.1 Indications

The main indications for SCS are now well established and comprise essentially ischaemic and neuropathic pain. SCS does not influence nociceptive (e.g. arthritic and acute post-operative) pain. The results in neuropathic pain are not as good as they are in ischaemia and some neuropathic syndromes respond better than others (Box 14.1). It should be remembered that SCS is not the only form of neurostimulation available; cases that do not respond adequately might respond to peripheral nerve, sacral root, or brain stimulation.

Box 14.1 Indications for spinal cord stimulation

Good indications
- Angina
- Peripheral vascular disease (obstructive and vasospastic)
- Complex regional pain syndrome
- Neuropathic limb pain following spinal surgery ('failed back or neck surgery syndrome')
- Peripheral nerve damage
- Brachial plexus damage (not avulsion)

Intermediate indications
- Amputation pain (stump pain better than phantom pain)
- Axial pain following spinal surgery
- Intercostal neuralgia
- Spinal cord (partial) damage

Poor indications
- Supraspinal central pain
- Perineal and anorectal pain

Not indicated
- Complete spinal cord transection
- Nerve root avulsion
- Non-ischaemic nociceptive pain.

Although it has long been known that SCS can stabilize the hyperexcitable neurogenic bladder, the exciting prospect has only very recently emerged that visceral pain, such as in severe irritable bowel syndrome and oesophageal spasm, and pancreatic and chronic post-laparotomy pain, may also respond to SCS. The neuropathic element of these conditions and others, e.g. interstitial cystitis, is now increasingly recognized; autonomic dysfunction is of course a feature of several of the more established indications of SCS.

14.3.2 **Other considerations**

There are very few contraindications (Box 14.2). Case selection is crucially important and the diagnosis alone is insufficient; it is not understood why patients with the same favourable diagnosis (see Box 14.1) may respond differently. Trial stimulation via temporary external connections is not a complete solution. Even when conducted thoroughly over a month or more, the resulting long-term success rate in neuropathic pain rarely exceeds 65–70%. The one-in-three failure rate reflects both the clinical complexity of many patients with neuropathic pain and the methodology of trial stimulation (see Assessment of outcome, p.131). Trials do not effectively exclude placebo responders and desperate wishful thinkers, but may exclude others who would obtain a useful effect in the long term but who do not attain the arbitrary pass mark.

Appraisal by a psychologist has not been shown to improve the success rate overall, but it does provide an important opportunity for detailed assessment and counselling. Patients' expectations must be appropriate: complete abolition of the pain should not be expected, although it can occur; in mixed syndromes any nociceptive element will not respond; a favourable modification of the pain should permit a reduction or cessation of medication and improved activity with concomitant increase in the ability to cope with any residual pain. SCS will not by itself, however, convert a miserable life into a rewarding one.

Box 14.2 **Contraindications to spinal cord stimulation**

Absolute
- Demand-type cardiac pacemaker
- Implanted cardiac defibrillator
- Uncontrolled coagulopathy
- Sepsis

Relative
- Cognitive impairment

14.4 **Equipment and methodology**

14.4.1 **Electrode placement**

The electrodes are placed in the posterior epidural space by one of two methods. 'Wire' or 'catheter' systems can be inserted percutaneously via a Tuohy needle, usually under local anaesthesia. This is minimally invasive, allows feedback to optimize the positioning, and the implanter does not have to be a surgeon. On the negative side these systems usually cannot penetrate epidural scarring (but can penetrate the dura), are electrically inefficient, and are more prone to dislodgement than are the alternative plate electrodes. The latter require an open operation and are often referred to as 'surgical' electrodes or leads. They are more efficient and more secure and there is some evidence that they are more effective, but their insertion usually requires a general anaesthetic and entails a bigger procedure (Fig. 14.1).

Both rostrocaudal and lateral positioning of the electrodes determine the distribution of the evoked paraesthesiae. Four available contacts have long been the norm (Fig. 14.2) and dual-channel technology greatly increases the versatility by allowing electronic 'steering'. More complex systems give even more flexibility.

Fig 14.1 Percutaneously implantable (left) and surgical (right) electrode systems for spinal cord stimulation. (Courtesy of Advanced Bionics, Inc.)

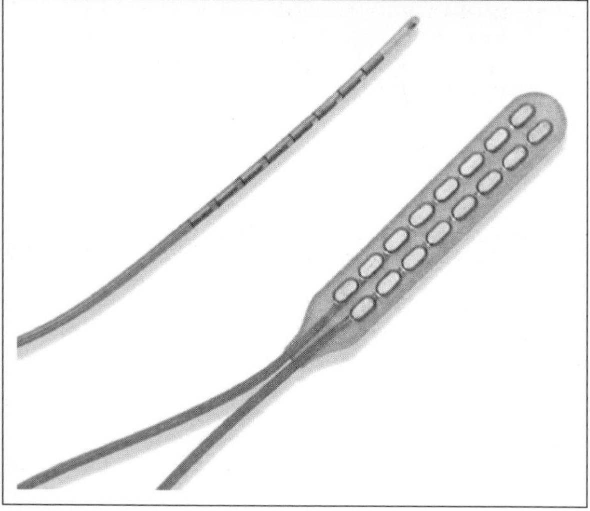

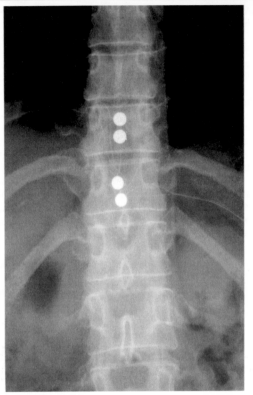

Fig 14.2 Radiograph showing four-contact plate electrode system (Lamitrode-22 ™; Advanced Neuromodulation Systems Inc.) in the lower thoracic spine

14.4.2 **Power sources**

The power source can be either an implanted pulse generator (IPG) similar to a cardiac pacemaker (Fig. 14.3) or an external transmitter linked to an internal receiver-transducer by radiofrequency (RF) coupling from an antenna on the skin. The former is less cumbersome but the power source will become depleted after an average of about five or six years (newer devices may last longer) depending on usage; surgical replacement will then be required, which also represents a significant recurring cost. Rechargeable systems have very recently become available and may obviate the need for RF systems.

IPGs are programmed by telemetry to adjust frequency, pulse width and amplitude, selection of contacts and their polarity, plus various cycling options. The patient has a home programmer to select pre-set programmes and adjust the amplitude. RF transmitters can be similarly programmed.

The relatively high initial cost belies the increasingly well-established cost-effectiveness with break-even occurring by three years.

14.5 Assessment of outcome

14.5.1 Assessment measures
It might be assumed that assessing the effect of SCS in neuropathic pain would be straightforward. In some clearly successful cases it is, but in many others the clinical complexity, including the effects of long-term pain, long-term disability, and long-term medication, confuses the issue. The confusion is compounded by inappropriate reliance on numerical rating scales of pain intensity, by the difference between clinical and statistical significance, by the influence of memory, by the natural variability over time, and by the lack of a meaningful definition of success (50% reduction in pain is not meaningful in a long-term condition). Some of these flaws also affect trial stimulation (see above).

14.5.2 Evidence of benefit
For the treatment as a whole there is very little class I evidence. There are only two randomized controlled trials with appropriate follow-up periods, one for reflex sympathetic dystrophy, now known as CRPS type I, and one for failed back surgery syndrome. More are needed but the outcome measures used must be appropriate and holistic.

Fig 14.3 Implantable, programmable pulse generator for therapeutic neurostimulation. (Courtesy of Advanced Bionics, Inc.)

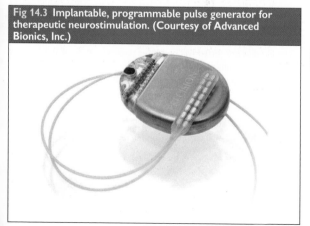

> **Box 14.3 Complications and other adverse considerations**
>
> **Complications**
> - Infection (2–5%)
> - Dural puncture (percutaneous leads)
> - Epidural haematoma (rare)
> - Permanent neurological damage (very rare)
> - Lead migration (commoner with percutaneous than plate electrodes and in the cervical spine)
> - Lead fracture
> - Failure of other components
>
> **Drawbacks/warnings**
> - Cannot generally undergo magnetic resonance imaging (MRI)
> - Cannot receive therapeutic diathermy
> - Special precautions with surgical diathermy
> - Cannot drive with stimulator switched on
> - Triggering security systems (carry an ID card or bracelet)

Unlike medication, SCS has virtually no side-effects. It does of course have risks, complications, and disadvantages (Box 14.3) and should be practised by experienced multidisciplinary teams. Difficulties aside, delivering significant benefit in up to 70% of appropriately selected patients for whom nothing else has been effective makes SCS a very useful treatment.

14.6 **The future**

- Devices will become more sophisticated but some of the requirements – versatility, reliability, small size, longevity, and low cost – may be mutually exclusive.
- The conditions treated will be better understood, e.g. CRPS, thereby improving case selection.
- Both case selection and outcome assessment will improve.
- New indications (e.g. visceral pain) will be established.
- Earlier implementation may modify disease natural history, rather than simply palliating.
- More high-quality clinical and scientific research will be published.

Key references

Kemler, M.A., De Vet, H.C., Barendse, G.A., Van Den Wildenberg, F.A., and Van Kleef, M. (2004). The effect of spinal cord stimulation in patients with chronic reflex sympathetic dystrophy: two years' follow-up of the randomized controlled trial. *Ann. Neurol.*, **55**, 13–18.

Melzack, R. and Wall, P.D. (1965). Pain mechanisms: a new theory. *Science*, **150**, 971–9.

North, R.B., Kidd, D.H., Farrokhi, F. and Piantadosi, S.A. (2005). Spinal cord stimulation versus repeated lumbosacral spine surgery for chronic pain: a randomized, controlled trial. *Neurosurgery*, **56**, 98–107.

Simpson, B.A., (ed.) (2003). *Electrical stimulation and the relief of pain.* Elsevier, Amsterdam.

Simpson, K. and Stannard, C. (ed.) (2005). *Spinal cord stimulation for the management of pain: recommendations for best clinical practice.* British Pain Society, London.

Chapter 15

Intrathecal drug delivery and neurolytic blocks

Karen H. Simpson and Vivienne Barros D'Sa

> ### Key points
>
> - Intrathecal drug delivery allows drugs to be placed nearer to central receptors and drug side-effects may be reduced because small doses are required compared to systemic administration.
> - External or internal intrathecal delivery systems are available and should only be implanted following careful patient selection.
> - Opioids, local anaesthetics, and clonidine are the most commonly used intrathecal drugs, though newer drugs such as ziconotide show promise.
> - Neurolytic blocks are usually confined to neuropathic pain arising from cancer or peripheral vascular disease. Coeliac plexus block for upper abdominal cancer pain, or lumbar sympathectomy for ischaemic leg pain, can be very effective.
> - Intracerebroventricular drug delivery is confined to neuropathic head pain, usually due to cancer. It is rarely used.

15.1 Intrathecal drug delivery

15.1.1 Background evidence

Intrathecal drug delivery (ITDD) allows drugs to be placed nearer to central receptors. Small drug doses are required compared to systemic administration and so drug side-effects may be reduced. ITDD was pioneered for cancer pain, but it is an alternative for persistent non-cancer neuropathic pains, e.g. plexus avulsions, amputation pain, vascular pain, and radicular pain, in which uncontrolled outcome studies have suggested benefits.

Uncertainties about selection often weaken trial results; long-term, randomized controlled trial (RCT) evidence supporting ITDD is lacking. Many studies do not assess the important functional aspects of the neuropathic pain experience. A study of patients with severe pain who were selected for ITDD showed that they improved with the therapy over 36 months, but their overall severity of pain and symptoms remained high. When patients with back and leg pain were assessed a year after ITDD, pain ratings improved by 47% (back pain) and 31% (leg pain – probably the neuropathic component); over 65% had reduced disability scores and at 12 months, 80% ITDD patients were satisfied with therapy. In a study that compared the efficacy and cost-effectiveness of ITDD with that of conventional therapy for pain from failed back surgery syndrome over five years, there was a 27% improvement of patients' disability in the ITDD group, compared with 12% in the control group. The high initial costs of ITDD were recovered by 28 months, and conventional therapy became relatively more expensive.

15.1.2 Practical considerations

ITDD should only be considered if simpler, safer, and more economical methods of analgesia provide inadequate benefits. Patients must be carefully selected to ensure that ITDD is appropriate (Box 15.1). An intrathecal (IT) test dose of the proposed medication(s)

Box 15.1 Indications and contraindications to ITDD

Indications

- Systemic analgesia effective, intolerable side-effects
- Good response to test dose
- Favourable psychosocial evaluation
- Multidisciplinary team experienced with ITDD
- Appropriate links to primary and other secondary care teams

Contraindications

- Patient refusal
- Head pain (often better managed by intracerebroventricular drug delivery)
- Inadequate analgesia or intolerable side-effects from test dose
- Poor patient concordance with ITDD
- Systemic infection (care with diabetic, immune suppressed, and neutropenic patients)
- Localized infection in sites of potential surgery
- Non-correctable coagulopathy
- Raised intracranial pressure
- Impending spinal cord compression
- Allergy to proposed intrathecal medication or implantable devices
- Lack of support services for ongoing care

may predict whether implantation is indicated. There are differences in response to bolus injection and infusion, so testing requires careful assessment. Using the epidural route for testing may be unhelpful as some drugs do not cross the dura readily, and dose equivalence is unclear. ITDD must be performed under full asepsis with fluoroscopic guidance; catheters should be placed posterior to the cord to reduce the granuloma risk. General anaesthesia may be needed, especially in children or if pain prevents positioning of the patient. The main infection risk seems to correlate with procedure duration, so it is important that experienced teams are involved.

ITDD is invasive and there are risks of procedure, equipment-related, and drug-related complications that must be explained to patients and their carers (Table 15.1). ITDD is a long-term commitment for the patient and the health care teams.

Table 15.1 Complications of ITDD (Always check for causes not related to ITDD)

Complication	Management
Procedure related	
Post-spinal headache	Keep patient lying down, standard analgesics and IV fluids? Autologous epidural blood patch
Total spinal	Aggressive resuscitation
Bleeding	Clinical observation for spinal compression – magnetic resonance imaging (MRI) and alert surgeon early
Neural damage to spinal cord/nerve roots	MRI early and surgical referral
Infection	Prevent infection with strict stand unit protocols
	Single dose of prophylactic antibiotics
	No evidence to support post-procedure antibiotics
	Suspected infection, hospitalization, infection screen, microbiologist advice, aggressive anti-microbials
Superficial wound infection	Frequent observation, antibiotics
Pump pocket seroma	If infected, intravenous (IV) antibiotics
	Removal of the system may be required
Infection of catheter or implant pocket	Remove system, IV antibiotics
Meningitis	Remove system, IV antibiotics
Epidural abscess	MRI, alert a surgeon, remove system, IV antibiotics

Table 15.1 Contd.	
Complication	Management
Drug related* – immediate	
Nausea and vomiting	Anti-emetics
Urinary retention	Intermittent catheterization
Pruritis	Antihistamines, ondansetron
Ventilatory depression	Naloxone
Confusion	Review systemic and ITDD doses, change IT drug choice
Drug related – delayed	
Myoclonus	Change from opioids or use systemic benzodiazepines
Oedema	Change from opioids
Arthralgia	
Facial flushing	
Sweating	Systemic low-dose clonidine
Constipation	Bowel care
Suppressed hypothalamic-pituitary axis	Monitor endocrine function and replacement treatments
(* complications depend on drug used)	
Equipment related	
Allergy to equipment	May require removal of system
Catheter related	
• Obstruction of tip or catheter	Flush system under radiological screening, may need surgical correction
• Catheter sheer, damage and/or spinal fluid leak	Manage headache, may need surgery
• Catheter tip granulomas	MRI, surgical decompression, and re-moval of mass/catheter
Pump failure, refill or programming error	
• Over dose	Stop pump and manage drug effects
• Under dose	Check pump, replacement drug therapy

15.1.3 ITDD systems

External systems are most appropriate for patients with a relatively short life expectancy (<3–4 months) and for those who require larger-volume spinal infusions. The procedure is simple, systems may be implanted under either local or general anaesthesia, and recovery after implant is quick. The catheter is tunnelled subcutaneously away from the spine, usually to the abdomen. The system must have two antibacterial filters and remain closed. An external pump is used that should have a capacity of at least 250ml, give very low volume infusions with precision, be easy to programme and portable.

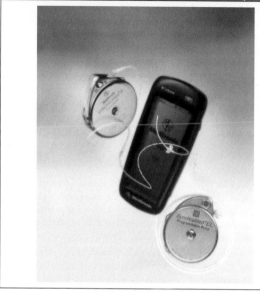

Fig 15.1 Examples of implantable intrathecal infusion devices (one with additional side port for bolus injections), and a telemetry programmer (Courtesy of Medtronic Inc.)

Internal pumps may be gas driven and deliver medication at a fixed rate, or battery driven (programmed via non-invasive telemetry); some of these programmable pumps allow patients to deliver boluses (Fig. 15.1). The 10–50ml pump is implanted into a subcutaneous pocket in the abdominal wall, often under general anaesthesia. It is refilled percutaneously, with strict asepsis. Programmable pumps are more expensive and need to be replaced when the battery fails, usually around seven to 10 years. All health care professionals involved, whether in primary or secondary care, must be trained on ITDD.

15.2 Intrathecal drugs

Many drugs have been given intrathecally, often almost empirically. Large-scale, long-term RCTs are needed to allow recommendations to be made about ITDD benefits and risks in patients with neuropathic pain. Drug selection needs to be refined and validated. Data about neurotoxicity of spinal drugs is important. Preservative-free formulations should be used and drug stability in delivery systems and spinal fluid should be considered. Combining drugs with different mechanisms of action can produce synergy that may reduce side-effects.

15.2.1 **Opioids**

Opioids should probably be first-line therapy. Low IT doses should be used, reducing systemic opioid and gradually titrating. Patients with neuropathic pain may require higher IT doses than patients with nociceptive pain, especially with monotherapy. Central side-effects are often greater with hydrophilic drugs than with lipophilic drugs. Other opioid-induced adverse effects include itch, peripheral oedema, urinary retention, and endocrine or immune complications. Switching IT opioids can sometimes restore efficacy and reduce side-effects.

15.2.2 **Local anaesthetics**

Local anaesthetics given with opioids may reduce opioid tolerance. Bupivacaine is commonly used; ropivacaine and levo-bupivacaine are less cardiotoxic, but there is little evidence that they are better than bupivacaine.

15.2.3 **Clonidine**

Clonidine has a synergistic effect with opioids (see Chapter 16), and can be a useful adjunct to spinal opioids for those with neuropathic pain; it may cause sedation, bradycardia, and hypotension. Severe rebound hypertension can occur with abrupt cessation of IT clonidine. Animal models and case reports suggest that spinal clonidine (<50µg daily) may enhance analgesia from spinal cord stimulation (SCS) in neuropathic pain.

15.2.4 **Baclofen**

Baclofen is a gamma amino butyric acid-B (GABA$_B$) agonist, used intrathecally for spasticity. Side-effects include muscle weakness and sedation. Low starting doses and slow titration are needed. Acute spinal baclofen withdrawal may lead to serious side-effects; deaths have been reported. Baclofen is analgesic in animals at doses below those needed for muscle relaxation. IT baclofen has been beneficial in some clinical refractory neuropathic pains, e.g. complex regional pain syndrome and central pain after stroke. There is synergy with other IT drugs and it has been used as an adjunct to SCS.

15.2.5 **Ziconotide**

Intrathecal ziconotide is a highly selective, potent, and reversible blocker of neuronal N-type voltage-sensitive calcium channels, with analgesic efficacy. It must be titrated very slowly over a number of weeks to minimize the adverse effects that were common in early studies due to fast titration and high dosing. Adverse effects at higher doses include dizziness, blurred vision, nystagmus, sedation, and psychomimetic effects. There is little tolerance after prolonged use. Ziconotide has a favourable risk/benefit ratio with advantages over several currently available IT therapies for pain, but RCTs are awaited.

15.2.6 **Ketamine**

Ketamine, a non-competitive *N*-methyl D-aspartate (NMDA) receptor antagonist, alters pain perception at spinal level. Concerns about toxicity after neuraxial use of racemic ketamine have led to the IT use of the preservative-free active compound, S (+)-ketamine (see also Chapter 11). Cases of severe neuropathic cancer pain have been treated successfully by IT infusion of morphine, bupivacaine, clonidine, and S (+)-ketamine. However, there are no pre-clinical safety data. Post-mortem observation of the spinal cord and nerve roots in some cases revealed histological abnormalities. Therefore neuraxial administration of S (+)-ketamine cannot be recommended for clinical practice without more data.

15.2.7 **Other drugs**

Animal work demonstrated a role for spinal benzodiazepines in regulating nociception. Midazolam has been given IT in clinical situations, despite concerns about pre-clinical safety data. At present there are no RCTs to support its use.

Animal models also provide insights into future IT therapies. Melatonin agonists can reduce the generation, development, and maintenance of central sensitization in neuropathic pain models. Nerve growth factor reverses neuropathic pain symptoms and restores opioid efficacy in animal models of neuropathic pain.

15.3 **Neurolytic blocks**

15.3.1 **Background**

Neurolysis in the peripheral nervous system has been replaced by other strategies, as it is unlikely to produce long-lasting analgesia and may lead to deafferentation pain. However, neurolytic blocks are useful in some patients with trigeminal neuralgia, cancer, or ischaemic vascular conditions, when pain is often fully or partly neuropathic.

Neurolytic sympathetic plexus blocks (NSPB) can relieve pain and improve quality of life in cancer patients. A study of 60 patients with abdominal or pelvic cancer pain (in two different disease phases) compared NSPB with pharmacological therapy alone, over eight weeks. Those who had NSPB early and later in their disease had a significant reduction of pain and opioid consumption, and a better quality of life than those who were pharmacologically managed. Opioid-related adverse effects were significantly greater in the drug-treated group. Occasional complications were transitory. NSPB for the management of cancer pain should be considered earlier in the disease, and calls into question the World Health Organization recommendations of using blocks as a last resort.

Patients must be carefully assessed and investigated to determine whether or not a nerve block is feasible and likely to help. The procedure and its benefits and burdens must be explained to the patient. Radiological imaging, with or without contrast, is helpful for some blocks and mandatory for others, e.g. coeliac plexus block. A temporary local anaesthetic block may predict the response to a neurolytic block. The use of nerve blocks as prognostic tools can be difficult because of confounding factors, e.g. systemic absorption of local anaesthetics leading to analgesia and placebo response.

15.3.2 Trigeminal blocks

Microvascular decompression via posterior fossa craniotomy, percutaneous gasserian glycerol neurolysis, balloon compression, and radiofrequency trigeminal lesion can all be used to treat trigeminal neuralgia that is resistant to medical therapy. These ganglion-level interventions are more effective than peripheral procedures, but no approach can be totally relied on to produce long-term pain relief. All of these techniques are neurodestructive and can cause sensory loss and dysaesthesia. At longer follow-up intervals, microvascular decompression is predicted to be the most cost-effective procedure, and should be considered the preferred operation for patients if their risk for general anaesthesia is acceptable. Percutaneous surgery may be better for older patients with medically unresponsive trigeminal neuralgia.

15.3.3 Lumbar sympathectomy

Interruption of the lumbar sympathetic chain can provide pain relief for some patients with vascular neuropathic pain, e.g. non-reconstructable critical leg ischaemia. Pre-operative ankle-brachial index has prognostic value, with clinical improvement if it is >0.3. Diabetes, angiography, palpable popliteal pulses, age, and sex are not predictive; results are not as good in smokers. Patients with rest pain alone do better than those with gangrene, especially of the big toe. Once gangrene is more extensive then sympathectomy is probably not helpful for limb salvage, but may help neuropathic pain and stump healing.

When considering non-vascular neuropathic pain, e.g. complex regional pain syndrome, the use of sympathectomy in clinical practice is based on very weak evidence (see Chapter 7). Some animal data has suggested that sympathectomy is effective when the animals show severe mechanical hypersensitivity, but more detailed clinical research is needed. Complications include: postural hypotension (especially if bilateral block is performed), genito-femoral neuritis, sexual dysfunction, renal damage, lumbar plexus damage, injection into the aortic wall leading to dissection, and intraperitoneal, epidural, or intrathecal injection.

15.3.4 Coeliac plexus block (CPB) and superior hypogastric plexus block (SHPB)

Coeliac plexus block (CPB) can provide good pain relief in some visceral pains that may be associated with visceral hyperalgesia, and thus be considered as partly neuropathic. CPB is used for patients with pain from upper abdominal cancer, and superior hypogastric plexus block (SHPB) for cancer pain arising from the pelvis and perineum. The role of neurolytic sympathetic blocks in advanced cancer, when pain syndromes may involve other structures, e.g. posterior abdominal and pelvic walls, is less clear. There are several different approaches to CPB, including retro-crural, trans-crural, trans-aortic, anterior, and greater splanchnic nerve block; complications can occur (Box 15.2). In a survey of 36 patients with advanced pancreatic or pelvic cancer pain, a neuropathic component was more common in those with pelvic cancers. These patients had less pain relief after neurolytic blocks than patients with pain due to pancreatic cancer.

Box 15.2 Complications of coeliac plexus block

- Local pain
- Diarrhoea
  - Usually resolves within 48 hours (if not consider octreotide)
- Hypotension
  - Usually resolves within 48 hours
  - Use adequate hydration and support stockings
  - Vasopressors occasionally needed
- Neurological complications
  - Lower extremity weakness and paraesthesia
  - Lumbar plexus damage
  - Epidural placement of neurolytic agent
  - Lumbar puncture
  - Urinary or faecal incontinence
  - Sexual dysfunction
  - Paraplegia
- Significant non-neurological adverse effects
  - Pneumothorax
  - Shoulder, chest, and pleuritic pain
  - Hiccup
  - Haematuria
  - Aortic dissection
  - Silent gastric perforation

15.3.5 Intrathecal neurolytic injection of sacrococcygeal nerve roots

Intrathecal neurolysis was commonly used for unilateral pain in the thoracic and lumbar area. Serious adverse effects such as motor blockade are possible, and now with the advent of spinal drug delivery, this technique is not used commonly. However, it still has value in the management of some cancer pain problems, e.g. pelvic and perineal pain.

15.4 Intracerebroventricular drug delivery (ICVDD)

Drugs can be delivered directly into the cerebral ventricles; this requires a surgical transcranial approach, with its accompanying morbidity. Intracerebroventricular drug delivery (ICVDD) can be useful for those with neuropathic head pain, usually due to cancer. Uncontrolled studies suggest that ICVDD is at least as effective as other neuraxial treatments, and may be successful for patients whose pain is resistant to other therapies.

Key references

Abram, S.E. (2000). Neural blockade for neuropathic pain. *Clin. J. Pain*, **16**, S56–61.

Ballantyne, J.C. and Carwood, C.M. (2005). Comparative efficacy of epidural, subarachnoid, and intra-cerebroventricular opioids in patients with pain due to cancer. *Cochrane Database of Systematic Reviews*, Issue 1; CD005178.

Hicks, F. and Simpson, K.H. (2004). *Nerve blocks in palliative care*. Oxford University Press, Oxford.

Mailis, A. and Furlan, A. (2003). Sympathectomy for neuropathic pain. *Cochrane Database of Systematic Reviews*, Issue 2; CD002918.

Prager, J.P. (2002). Neuraxial medication delivery: the development and maturity of a concept for treating chronic pain of spinal origin. *Spine*, **27**, 2593–605.

Chapter 16

Drug synergy and sequencing

Michael I. Bennett

Key points

- Combinations of drugs that work through different mechanisms can result in additive or synergistic effects that may improve control of pain, reduce side-effects, or both.
- Most evidence comes from studies of co-analgesics with opioids and is derived from both animal and clinical research.
- Although number needed to treat (NNT) is used to compare drug effectiveness, this method may miss some benefits, overestimate reliability (if confidence intervals are wide), and may detract from number needed to harm (NNH).
- Stepwise or parallel approaches to drug combinations have equal merit.
- First-line approaches can be initiated in primary care but second- and third-line approaches will require increasingly close liaison with specialist pain management services.

16.1 Rationale for combination treatment

16.1.1 Drug synergy

In neuropathic pain, the main purpose of utilizing drug combinations is to improve pain control and reduce adverse effects. By combining drugs with different mechanisms of action, additive or even synergistic analgesic effects can be achieved whilst minimizing adverse effects. This results in better pain control and improved concordance with drug treatment.

Drug synergy is produced when the effects of a drug combination are greater than when the individual drug effects are simply added together. In other words, synergy is a situation where one plus one equals three. Demonstrating synergy in clinical practice can be difficult but as an example, if 1mg of drug A plus 1mg of drug B results in the same effect as 5mg of drug A or drug B alone, then synergy is taking place. If the combination results in the same effect as 2mg of A or B alone, then the effects are additive, not synergistic.

There are two broad types of drug synergy based on the nature of the interaction: pharmacodynamic or pharmacokinetic. Pharmacodynamic synergy results from two drugs with different actions directed at a similar target or physiological system. A good example of this is the use of rifampicin and isoniazid in the treatment of tuberculosis. Pharmacokinetic synergy results when one drug influences the absorption, distribution, biotransformation, or elimination of another drug. A classic example of this is the combination of amoxicillin with clavulanic acid; the latter prevents the breakdown of the former by beta-lactamase producing bacteria.

16.1.2 **Evidence from pre-clinical studies**

Animal studies have shown powerful evidence for short term (hours or days) drug synergy in neuropathic pain. In these studies, differences in mechanisms of action of individual analgesic drugs are exploited and their neurochemical and physiological effects can be studied in great detail. For example, sub-anti-nociceptive doses of intrathecal morphine (i.e. doses that do not prevent the sensation of pain) are enhanced when combined with oral gabapentin. This anti-nociceptive effect is reversed by naloxone, suggesting that the effects are not directly related to gabapentin. Instead gabapentin appears to enhance the action of morphine at μ opioid receptors, a pharmacodynamic synergy. This implies that lower doses of morphine combined with gabapentin can be used to produce the same effects when compared to morphine alone.

Other studies have also revealed useful insights into the effects of drug combinations in neuropathic pain. A combination of an opioid (either morphine or methadone) with the N-methyl D-aspartate (NMDA) antagonist ketamine has been given either alone or in combination to rats with a mononeuropathy (caused by ligating the sciatic nerve to produce neuropathic pain). When the neuropathic paw and a normal paw were exposed to pressure testing, synergistic effects were only apparent in the neuropathic paw and not the normal paw. This demonstrates that the opioid–ketamine combination is most effective in the presence of hyperexcitability associated with neuropathic pain, rather than in the context of nociceptive pain.

16.2 **Drug combinations in clinical practice**

The great majority of clinical trials have been conducted with combinations of an opioid and a co-analgesic.

16.2.1 **Opioids with tricyclics**

Tricyclic antidepressants have been studied extensively in the context of neuropathic pain. Amitriptyline has been found to increase plasma morphine through inhibition of hepatic glucuronidation. This potentially allows lower doses of morphine to be given with amitriptyline for the same or better analgesic effect than if morphine is given alone, a pharmacokinetic synergy. Amitriptyline also results in increased expression of leu-enkephalin, a naturally occurring opioid within the central nervous system, which can mimic therapeutic opioid effects. These findings have given rise to the idea that tricyclics are 'opioid sparing'.

A recent clinical trial in patients with post-herpetic neuralgia provides good evidence for using combinations of opioid with tricyclic antidepressants. In this study, patients were entered into a randomized crossover of opioid (morphine or methadone), tricyclic (nortriptyline or desipramine), and placebo. Active drugs reduced pain much more than placebo, as expected. However, patients who experienced good relief with opioid didn't necessarily experience good relief with tricyclics, and vice versa. Although the study did not directly examine the effects of a combination of opioid and tricyclic, it did clearly demonstrate that the active drugs produce analgesia through different mechanisms, suggesting the potential for a pharmacodynamic synergy.

16.2.2 **Opioids with anti-epileptics**

Although animal studies have shown a synergistic effect between morphine and gabapentin, clinical evidence in patients has been lacking until recently. A well-designed trial compared the effects of morphine, gabapentin, a combination of both, and placebo in patients with painful diabetic neuropathy or post-herpetic neuralgia. Patients were treated with each arm for five weeks at a time. The final analysis revealed that morphine and gabapentin produced similar analgesic benefits (morphine was slightly better), but the combination resulted in significantly greater analgesia than either drug alone. In fact, the combination consisted of much lower doses of either drug than when used alone. Adverse effects of this combination consisted of constipation, sedation, and dry mouth.

16.2.3 **Opioids with NMDA antagonists**

Two drugs with activity at the NMDA receptor have been studied in combination with opioids: ketamine and dextromethorphan (see also

Chapter 11). When ketamine was given alongside morphine in a small study of cancer patients, whose pain was previously unrelieved by morphine alone, almost all experienced additional analgesic benefit. Adverse effects were frequent, but may reflect the frailty of the patients in the study.

Dextromethorphan has received more attention recently as an NMDA receptor antagonist. It has been combined with morphine in a 1:1 ratio to examine whether it can enhance analgesia or prevent tolerance to chronic opioid administration. Trials lasting around four weeks in a group of patients with mixed cancer and non-cancer pain types (nociceptive, neuropathic) showed that patients receiving the combination needed only half the dose of morphine to achieve good pain control compared to the morphine-only group. Interestingly, a longer trial of three months in non-neuropathic-pain patients failed to show an advantage of the combination over morphine alone. Whether this reflects the fact that any advantage wears off in the longer term, that the amount of dextromethorphan was too low, or that the combination is only effective in the presence of hyperexcitability (see above) is not known. Very soon, phase three trials will begin of a combination of dextromethorphan with an enzyme inhibitor that slows the drug's rapid metabolism in the liver.

16.2.4 Opioids and cholecystokinin antagonists

Cholecystokinin (CCK) antagonists such as proglumide (see Chapter 10) are known to mediate opioid tolerance in animal models and have been examined in clinical trials. Proglumide has been shown to enhance opioid analgesia, when combined with dihydrocodeine or morphine, in cancer and non-cancer pain. Although these patients did not have exclusive neuropathic pain, this evidence suggests that synergistic effects occur with this combination that may be applicable to neuropathic pain.

16.2.5 Intrathecal opioids with local anaesthetic or clonidine

In cases of neuropathic pain that require intrathecal drug delivery (see Chapter 15), combination treatment is often used. Clinical trial evidence clearly supports the addition of clonidine to opioid in this context to enhance analgesia. Local anaesthetic drugs have also been found to enhance opioid analgesia and reduce the development of tolerance. The mechanisms through which these effects occur are not clear.

16.3 **Drug sequencing: stepwise or parallel approaches?**

16.3.1 **A word about NNT and NNH**

The array of drugs that have been examined in neuropathic pain is wide and supported by varying levels of evidence from small case reports to large randomized controlled trials. Condensing this information into a clinically useful management strategy is not easy but is helped by the use of the concepts of number needed to treat (NNT) and number needed to harm (NNH). These respectively refer to the number of patients that need to be treated for one to experience significant pain relief, or significant harm, in comparison with a placebo arm (see also Chapter 9). Significant pain relief is usually taken to mean a reduction in pain score by at least 50%; however, systematic reviews have included trials where 'excellent' or 'good' pain relief occurred (without numerical data), and sometimes 'moderate' pain relief. These different definitions of success will impact on the apparent effectiveness or otherwise of a drug. Also, these analyses may miss important information because they rely on bimodal yes or no criteria.

Recently, a 30% reduction in pain has been demonstrated to be a meaningful benefit for chronic pain patients. Using this less stringent threshold may alter the NNT value of analgesics in future, though evidence to date suggests that using either 30% or 50% threshold gives similar results. No trials have examined improved function as an outcome measure and some analgesics may allow greater activity for the same level of pain. Focusing on pain intensity alone may miss other benefits.

Also important are the confidence intervals (CI) that accompany a derived NNT; wide 95% CI suggest that the NNT has been derived from studies with few patients or that the drug itself has inconsistent effects. Remember also that NNT only tells one side of the story; NNH is also important. Ideally, a drug should have a NNT close to 1 (meaning that almost everyone who is treated experiences significant benefit) and a NNH that is very high (a large majority do not get adverse effects).

It has been argued that earlier studies of treatments in neuropathic pain may have been less able to detect and report adverse events. This would lead to an overestimation of NNH for older antiepileptics and tricyclic antidepressants when compared with more recent studies of co-analgesics, i.e. they appear better tolerated than is the case in clinical practice.

16.3.2 **Benefits and burdens of different approaches**

Stepwise treatment allows a clear relationship between a drug and its beneficial or adverse effects to be established. Patient concordance with medication is likely to be greater and treatment failure allows a drug to be discontinued before a second drug is introduced. This is important in situations where patients are taking medication for other co-morbid conditions and reduces the well-described risks of polypharmacy.

On the other hand, a parallel approach offers the chance of greater pain relief at lower drug doses with potentially fewer adverse effects. Initiating combination therapy may also reduce the time it takes to reach acceptable pain control compared to a stepwise approach. However, combination treatments may result in unpredictable adverse effects either through drug interactions (e.g. some anti-epileptics increase plasma levels of tricyclics) or because simultaneous titration of two drugs is more complicated than monotherapy. In addition, successful treatment with a combination approach does not exclude the fact that one drug in the combination may be redundant and/or contributing most of the adverse effects.

16.4 **A treatment algorithm**

There are no clinical trials that have tested a sequential approach to treating neuropathic pain. Based on the weight of evidence and experience in clinical practice, suggested approaches to managing neuropathic pain are presented in Table 16.1 (see also Fig. 9.2, Chapter 9).

16.4.1 **First-line approaches**

A useful first-line approach would be a tricyclic antidepressant such as amitriptyline, or an anti-epileptic such as gabapentin, pregabalin, or oxcarbazepine. The NNTs for all these drugs are very similar, between 2 and 3.5, depending on the type of neuropathic pain condition. Two small studies have compared amitriptyline directly with gabapentin and have not demonstrated reliably that one is better than the other. Choosing on the basis of adverse effects is probably the best course; for example, amitriptyline would be appropriate for patients who prefer once-daily dosing, have poor sleep, and who are less prone to antimuscarinic effects. Failure on one class (tricyclic or anti-epileptic) after a four to six-week period of titration would suggest that a trial of the other is indicated. Some experts use low doses of both tricyclics and anti-epileptics as first-line treatment. Additional measures such as TENS, acupuncture, or paracetamol may help.

Table 16.1 Approaches to the management of neuropathic pain

	Monotherapy	Combinations	Additional measures
A. First-line [Referral to specialized pain management service *not necessary*]	Tricyclic antidepressant (TCA), e.g. amitriptyline Anti-epileptic (AE), e.g. gabapentin or pregabalin	Low-dose TCA+AE	Paracetamol TENS Acupuncture
B. Second-line [Referral to specialized pain management service *desirable*]	Capsaicin Lidocaine patch Tizanidine Clonidine Baclofen Alternative antidepressant (e.g. duloxetine) Opioid: tramadol, morphine, oxycodone (see local protocols)	Opioid with TCA or AE	Physiotherapy Occupational therapy
C. Third-line [Referral to specialized pain management service *essential*]	Alternative opioids Ketamine Neuromodulation	Ketamine plus opioid Intrathecal drug delivery	Above plus: Psychological assessment and support

16.4.2 **Second-line approaches**

A second-line step in this sequential approach, after separate trials of tricyclics and anti-epileptics, might involve a trial of topical measures such as lidocaine patch or capsaicin cream. Other measures such as baclofen or tizanadine may be used. Opioids such as morphine, buprenorphine, tramadol, or oxycodone may be helpful; the latter has a reported NNT of 2.5. It would be important to enter this step after reviewing the clinical diagnosis and ensuring adherence to local protocols (and liaison with local pain management service) for using opioids in non-cancer chronic pain (see Chapter 12). Opioids could replace or be added to either of the drug classes that were used first-line.

16.4.3 **Third-line approaches**

Patients with neuropathic pain that has not improved with initial (and better evidence-based) treatment require additional measures. At this stage, the involvement of a specialized pain management or palliative care service is essential. The use of drugs such as ketamine and alternative opioids, together with neuromodulation, may be undertaken in more specialized facilities that also have access to psychological assessment and support.

16.4.4 **Cancer neuropathic pain**

Treating neuropathic pain in cancer patients as opposed to non-cancer patients may sometimes require a modified approach when prescribing analgesics. The difference is related to the patient rather than pain (see Chapter 8). Cancer patients are more likely to be frail, exhibit a changing pain picture, and have additional renal, hepatic, or cognitive impairment. This means that toxicity may be reached before benefit and therefore the NNT may be higher and NNH may be lower for analgesics in this group. Cancer patients with neuropathic pain or mixed pain types are more likely to have commenced opioid analgesia, and co-analgesic drugs are often combined with opioids to achieve good pain control. A large observational study demonstrated the success of this approach. Early intervention with intrathecal therapy or neurolytic blocks for severe cases is often indicated.

Key references

Gilron, I., Bailey, J.M., Dongsheng, T., Holden, R.R., Weaver, D.F., and Houlden, R.L. (2005). Morphine, gabapentin, or their combination for neuropathic pain. *N. Engl. J. Med.*, **352**, 1324–34.

Grond, S., Radbruch, L., Meuser, T., Sabatowski, R., Loick, G., and Lehmann, K.A. (1999). Assessment and treatment of neuropathic cancer pain following WHO guidelines. *Pain*, **79**, 15–20.

Namaka, M., Gramlich, C.R., Ruhlen, D., Melanson, M., Sutton, I., and Major, J. (2004). A treatment algorithm for neuropathic pain. *Clinical Therapeutics*, **26**, 951–79.

Raja, S. N., Haythornthwaite, J.A., Pappagallo, M., Clark, M.R., Travison, T.G., Sabeen, S. *et al.* (2003). Opioids versus antidepressants in postherpetic neuralgia: a randomized, placebo-controlled trial. *Neurology*, **59**, 1015–21.

Chapter 17

Patient perspectives

S. José Closs

> ### Key points
>
> - The impact of neuropathic pain on quality of life has been under-researched and poorly understood though survey and focus group research is helping to gain better insights into what patients suffer.
> - Neuropathic pain results in significant sleep disturbance, fatigue, and low mood (that sometimes leads to suicidal ideation), and side-effects from drug treatment are common.
> - Patients with neuropathic pain report strained relationships with spouses and friends, and reduced ability to work and carry out social roles.
> - Within the wider society, patients with neuropathic pain want to have their pain reports believed, and want more accurate information and better support from health care professionals.
> - Quality of life for patients with neuropathic pain can be improved when existing and newer drugs form part of a multifaceted approach to care, rather than when used in isolation.

17.1 Introduction

17.1.1 Measuring impact on quality of life

Most of our knowledge about neuropathic pain is concerned with its diagnosis and treatment, usually pharmacological. Pain textbooks often provide brief information about the main clinical features of neuropathic pain, but few give a realistic indication of its impact on the lives of patients who suffer from it.

The bizarre nature and unpredictability of this pain may have an enormous negative impact on many aspects of quality of life, including physical, psychological, spiritual, social, and economic aspects of patients' lives. Some aspects have received more attention than others: for example physical and emotional functions can be measured with established scales such as the Brief Pain Inventory. Increasingly, quality of life is being recognized as important and scales such as the Nottingham Health Profile, SF-36, and the EuroQol (EQ-5D) are being used in studies of people with neuropathic pain.

17.1.2 Evidence from patient surveys

There are few large surveys of people with neuropathic pain, but available information suggests that the majority experience severe discomfort due to pain and report that the pain interferes with general activity, work, mood, sleep, and enjoyment of life (see also Chapter 3). For 126 Swedish patients the most bothersome symptoms resulting from the pain were difficulty sleeping (88%), lack of energy (86%), difficulty in concentrating (76%), and drowsiness (71%) (see Meyer-Rosberg et al.). These patients showed poorer physical and social functioning and mental health than the general population. Similarly, a later survey of 602 Swedish patients showed that neuropathic pain severity was associated with poorer quality-of-life scores (details of these surveys are referenced below).

These tidy epidemiological descriptions of the problems do not communicate what these issues mean at a personal level. This chapter aims to illustrate how some of the key aspects of neuropathic pain impact on the daily lives of individuals. These include quotes from real patients who participated in a qualitative study of the impact of neuropathic pain funded by the British Pain Society (see Appendix 1). The quotes have been selected to illustrate points of major importance to this group.

17.2 Physical and psychological impact

17.2.1 Sleep disturbance and fatigue

Probably the most common problem resulting from neuropathic pain is disrupted sleep. Getting off to sleep, finding a comfortable position, and being woken by pain during the night may all become routine:

> I've not had a full night's sleep in four years … the most I get is three, maybe four hours if I'm lucky.

Considerable physical, emotional, and cognitive efforts are required to live with persistent pain, and sleep loss makes these more difficult. Fatigue may reduce the ability to concentrate due to the distracting nature of pain, making it more difficult to engage with the outside world when actively dealing with the pain.

> … you can't ignore the whole thing; you can't function, you can't think, you can't concentrate …

17.2.2 Emotional and psychological changes

Some patients report distressing changes in their mood:

> It [the pain] has affected me where I am bad tempered ...
> abrupt, snappy, certain times I'm fine, but it doesn't last long ...
> and then I really feel horrible. And I think why did I do that, and
> that's what's happening at the moment, this frustration is causing
> me to change into probably a horrible person.

> ... don't start making out that I'm mentally ill, there's a reason
> that I'm depressed. ... I've lost all my hobbies. I used to play
> guitar, ride mountain bikes, all them things have changed – and
> work's gone, my home's gone. Of course I'm gonna be depressed,
> I'd be a bloody idiot if I wasn't.

Many express concern that their families will become unable or
unwilling to live with their negative emotions, and those who recog-
nize the changes in themselves may experience guilt about their
effect on their loved ones.

Clearly, those with persistent severe neuropathic pain have to
cope with negative changes in many aspects of their lives. Suicidal
ideation is not uncommon among the worst cases:

> I have no life whatsoever you know and I've tried topping myself
> ... I did try and I laid there just thinking about my grandson and I
> thought how can you do that, my only grandchild, I love him
> dearly and he's going to find out that his grandma committed
> suicide. So I just had glass after glass of salted water and I puked
> that much ...

17.2.3 The undesirable side-effects of drugs

For the most part, medication use is the primary method of attempt-
ing to deal with symptoms. This may include both prescription and
non-prescription drugs, and their effectiveness and side-effects are
highly variable:

> I find that if I don't take that [the amitriptyline], the next day I'm
> like anxious and I think something's going to happen, that fear of
> something happening, so I have to take them ... I don't know if
> it's helping me.

> I'm really lethargic, really slow until I get into the afternoon when I
> feel quite normal, and then I take the tablets again and I go back
> down.

Increased appetite and the consequent increase in weight as well as a reduced ability to concentrate may be additional problems for those taking gabapentin:

> It upsets me – I've got to do something about it. He said to me, 'Well it's a side-effect. Would you rather have the pain?' That's not the point. I'm changing, my body shape, I don't want to look the way I do.

> … when I first started taking it I'm thinking I can't concentrate. I couldn't read a book, I still can't read a book really … I had to make a decision at one point to sort of reduce the gabapentin a little bit and have more pain just to be able to … A bit more clarity, I won't say brilliant, but a little bit more clarity, yeah.

> I feel better now I'm not taking as much. But my concentration, that's something I really suffer with.

17.3 Impact of neuropathic pain on direct social functioning

17.3.1 The impact on family life

Relationships within families can become strained, where previously established roles change. The loss of masculinity or femininity and the inability to fulfill traditional roles such as protecting children or supporting ageing parents may produce considerable distress:

> Yes, it's a man thing, you've lost all that what men stand for, if you know what I mean. If my daughter gets into trouble, I'm not in a position now to go and sort it out.

> … having to ask my dad to come and do it for me, do you know what I mean, and that's just wrong in my eyes. My parents have been there for me all my life and they're at an age now where they should be able to take it easy and rely on their son occasionally to help them out with stuff, and I can't do it for them. They understand, but it doesn't make it any easier from my point of view …

Marital relationships may crumble or break down altogether:

> You know if you're just sort of laid in bed and he puts his hand on my hip to give me a cuddle or anything, I say 'don't touch me' because it's just, it's just I can't even put my own hand there. I certainly don't want anybody else's big hand on me … 'Don't touch me, but you've still got to love me.' [laugh] Strange isn't it? … And half of the time you're in so much pain you can't be bothered anyway.

> I and my husband split up and we'd been married 36 years. We split up because he couldn't stand it any more.

17.3.2 **The impact on social activities**

Social isolation tends to increase as time goes on and friends reduce the frequency of invitations because of the unpredictability of symptoms. Practical difficulties associated with the pain also inhibit social activities:

> Yeah, because they ask you out and you're in agony, and nine times out of ten you have to turn round and say 'I'm sorry, I can't make it.' So in the end they think 'what's the point?'

> ... before the accident, in the summer if it were a nice sunny day you'd just jump in the car and away you went. ... You can't do that anymore because you don't know what you're going to be like that day when you wake up ...

> And when I've got to go shopping ... I've got to ask someone, to have someone to lift, and they look at you as if to say 'Are you kidding me?' And, you know, and it's like I can't stand there explaining, I just need the help there and then, and it gets so frustrating.

17.3.3 **Ability to work**

Most patients report that they attempt to maintain work roles for as long as possible. However, the impact of neuropathic pain symptoms, sleep disruption, and muscle fatigue may have severe consequences. Those with employers willing to be flexible may fare better, but most of those with severe symptoms become resigned to the fact that a return to full-time work is unlikely:

> I want to go out to work ... One of the pain specialists I went to see over my claims said, 'Oh yeah, he's suitable for work, but he'd have to try and get a job where he could do an hour then clear off for a couple of hours to recover and then come back.' Oh come on, give me a break. Who's going to set you on to do that and pay you for it?

17.4 **Patients with neuropathic pain in the wider society**

17.4.1 **Having their pain reports believed and understood**

A common problem for those with neuropathic pain is being believed and being understood. The invisible nature of pain means that others are unaware of it, unless they have explicitly been told, and even then they may not believe or comprehend the nature and extent of the impact of pain on an individual. This applies to health care professionals, work colleagues, and family and friends. Many in this group express dissatisfaction with general practitioners (GPs) and pain specialists:

> ... what's annoying is the person you see is a bog standard GP who's got to make an assessment on something he's got absolutely no idea about. I understood what he was saying, there really was nothing they could do, and he said to me, 'Look, people have to cope with pain. Take some tablets and cope.' And at that point I were at my lowest you know, and I said, 'But I feel that I can't live with it.' ... If I hadn't have had my family, the way I felt that day I could have quite easily come home and ended it.

Getting friends to understand pain that they can't actually see is a difficulty for many:

> You find that people don't believe you a lot of the time, they can't see it so they don't think there's anything the matter with you.

> It's just people's off-the-cuff 'Just get on with it.' ... It's like, what? You wouldn't say that if I came in and I had a bloody leg missing or something. ... You wouldn't react like that if I came in and I had multiple sclerosis or if I had cancer. You don't say to them 'Just bloody get on with it and leave it.'

Not being believed can cause sufferers considerable frustration and may produce a loss of credibility, threatening their integrity. Distress may also result from the notion that psychological problems are the cause of their pain.

> ... everything was so painful ... and you get really a bit depressed with it, and then when you go ... they try and say there's nothing, so they thought it must be psychological and that was the biggest insult for me.

17.4.2 **Their need for accurate information and appropriate support**

Neuropathic pain is difficult to treat successfully, so many sufferers continually seek new treatments and better information:

> If I take something it's mainly because I've gone to my GP and said I want to try this, because I've been through medical books and I've searched through and thought 'Right, this says it controls muscle spasms and so on. I'll try popping some of them.' And I'll actually go, because it's not nice to go and have someone just say 'Well, go and crack on with it, just get on with it.'

The recent burgeoning of complementary therapies has provided a questionable array of interventions which provide hope for those with neuropathic pain:

> I've tried acupuncture, massage, healing. I've tried everything, because like, you would do. So I have tried quite a lot of alternatives and nothing helps-nothing seems to, it [the pain] seems to have it's own will, it comes and goes.

> I've got self-hypnotism books at home. I'm trying to hypnotize myself and I'm reading and I'm thinking this is just bloody ridiculous, but I still go through the whole book and still sit there for weeks on end. And I couldn't do it.

The lack of consensus between different clinicians is a concern for some, and there is a desire for a single diagnosis and varying amounts of clear information. When doctors disagree with one another the consequences for the patient can be very serious and disempowering:

> I don't know about you but I find that with the different people you see you get so many different opinions. ... you're swapping about and for me now I got finished in my job from Dr A in Derby [who] did a medical [for my job] and then ... they said you can't work anymore ... then Dr B at Leeds did the medical for my pension and said, 'Oh you should go to work.' So I lost my job and then I didn't get my pension, so I ended up with nothing, and all on the fact that two people in the same bloody jobs got different opinions.

17.4.3 Potential for improvements in care

It is difficult for health care professionals to help these patients without understanding the genuine unpleasantness of their symptoms and the resulting misery. These experiences are the reason why health care professionals, researchers, and pharmaceutical companies invest so much effort into improving treatments for neuropathic pain. Although the emphasis tends to be on developing new drugs, the content of this chapter suggests that there is scope for improving family and social support, as well as information provision, cognitive therapies, complementary therapies, and perhaps developing other innovative approaches to helping sufferers of chronic neuropathic pain.

Key references

Closs, S.J., Staples, V., Briggs, M., and Bennett, M.I. (2005, unpublished data). *A qualitative study of the experience and impact of neuropathic pain symptoms*. Final report for the British Pain Society, London.

McDermott, A.M., Toelle, T.R., Rowbotham, D.J., Schaefer, C.P., and Dukes, E.M. (2006). The burden of neuropathic pain: results from a cross-sectional survey. *Eur. J. Pain*, **10**, 127–35.

Meyer-Rosberg, K., Burckhardt, C.S., Huizar, K., Kvarnström, A., Nordfors, L., and Kristofferson, A. (2001). A comparison of the SF-36 and Nottingham Health Profile in patients with chronic neuropathic pain. *Eur. J. Pain*, **5**, 391–403.

Appendix 1

Useful links

British Pain Society
British Pain Society
21 Portland Place
London
W1B 1PY
UK
www.britishpainsociety.org
info@britishpainsociety.org

BPS website contains position statement on 'The use of drugs beyond licence in palliative care and pain management' plus accompanying patient information leaflet. BPS has also published guidelines on opioids in persistent non-cancer pain and spinal cord stimulation.

International Association for the Study of Pain (IASP)
IASP
111 Queen Anne Avenue N
Suite 501
Seattle
WA 98109-4955
USA
www.iasp-pain.org

American Pain Society
American Pain Society
4700 W Lake Avenue
Glenview
IL 60025
USA
www.ampainsoc.org
info@ampainsoc.org

Pain Relief Foundation
Pain Relief Foundation
Clinical Sciences Centre
University Hospital Aintree
Lower Lane
Liverpool
L9 7AL
UK
www.painrelieffoundation.org.uk
secretary@painrelieffoundation.org.uk

The Neuropathy Trust

The Neuropathy Trust
PO Box 26
Nantwich
Cheshire
CW5 5FP
UK
www.neurocentre.com
admin@neurocentre.com

The Neuropathy Association

The Neuropathy Association
60 E 42nd Street
Suite 942
New York
NY 10165
USA
www.neuropathy.org

Martindale Pharmaceuticals Ltd

Martindale Pharmaceuticals Ltd
Bampton Road
Harold Hill
Romford
Essex
RM3 8UG
UK

Tel: (+44) 01708 386660
Fax: (+44) 01708 384032

Palliative Care Formulary on-line

www.palliativedrugs.com

Neuropathic pain descriptor scales

Leeds Assessment of Neuropathic Symptoms and Signs (LANSS)

Bennett, M. (2001). The LANSS pain scale: the Leeds Assessment of Neuropathic Symptoms and Signs. *Pain*, 92, 147–57.

THE LANSS PAIN SCALE
Leeds Assessment of Neuropathic Symptoms and Signs

NAME_____ DATE_____

This pain scale can help to determine whether the nerves that are carrying your pain signals are working normally or not. It is important to find this out in case different treatments are needed to control your pain.

A. PAIN QUESTIONNAIRE

- Think about <u>how your pain has felt over the last week</u>.
- Please say whether any of the descriptions match your pain exactly.

1. **Does your pain feel like strange, unpleasant sensations in your skin? Words like 'pricking', 'tingling', 'pins and needles' might describe these sensations.**

   a) NO – My pain doesn't really feel like this.................................. (0)

   b) YES – I get these sensations quite a lot.. (5)

2. **Does your pain make the skin in the painful area look different from normal? Words like 'mottled' or 'looking more red or pink' might describe the appearance.**

   a) NO – My pain doesn't affect the colour of my skin..................... (0)

   b) YES – I've noticed that the pain does make my skin look different from normal.... (5)

3. **Does your pain make the affected skin abnormally sensitive to touch? Getting unpleasant sensations when lightly stroking the skin, or getting pain when wearing tight clothes might describe the abnormal sensitivity.**

   a) NO – My pain doesn't make my skin abnormally sensitive in that area.......... (0)

   b) YES – My skin seems abnormally sensitive to touch in that area..................... (3)

4. **Does your pain come on suddenly and in bursts for no apparent reason when you're still? Words like 'electric shocks', 'jumping', and 'bursting' describe these sensations.**

   a) NO – My pain doesn't really feel like this.. (0)

   b) YES – I get these sensations quite a lot.. (2)

5. **Does your pain feel as if the skin temperature in the painful area has changed abnormally? Words like 'hot' and 'burning' describe these sensations.**

   a) NO – I don't really get these sensations.. (0)

   b) YES – I get these sensations quite a lot.. (1)

B. SENSORY TESTING

Skin sensitivity can be examined by comparing the painful area with a contra-lateral or adjacent non-painful area for the presence of allodynia and an altered pinprick threshold (PPT).

1. ALLODYNIA

Examine the response to lightly stroking cotton wool across the non-painful area and then the painful area. If normal sensations are experienced in the non-painful site, but pain or unpleasant sensations (tingling, nausea) are experienced in the painful area when stroking, allodynia is present.

a) NO, normal sensation in both areas.. (0)

b) YES, allodynia in painful area only.. (5)

2. ALTERED PINPRICK THRESHOLD

Determine the pinprick threshold by comparing the response to a 23-gauge (blue) needle mounted inside a 2ml syringe barrel placed gently on to the skin in non-painful and then painful areas.

If a sharp pinprick is felt in the non-painful area, but a different sensation is experienced in the painful area, e.g. none/blunt only (raised PPT) or a very painful sensation (lowered PPT), an altered PPT is present.

If a pinprick is not felt in either area, mount the syringe onto the needle to increase the weight and repeat.

a) NO, equal sensation in both areas.. (0)

b) YES, altered PPT in painful area.. (3)

SCORING:

Add values in parentheses for sensory description and examination findings to obtain overall score.

TOTAL SCORE (maximum 24) ....

If score <12, neuropathic mechanisms are **unlikely** to be contributing to the patient's pain.

If score ≥12, neuropathic mechanisms are **likely** to be contributing to the patient's pain.

Self-report LANSS (S-LANSS)

Bennett, M.I., Smith, B.H., Torrance, N., and Potter, J. (2005). The S-LANSS score for identifying pain of predominantly neuropathic origin: validation for use in clinic and postal research. *J. Pain,* **6**, 149–58.

THE S-LANSS PAIN SCORE

Leeds Assessment of Neuropathic Symptoms and Signs (self-complete)

NAME _____ DATE _____

- This questionnaire can tell us about the type of pain that you may be experiencing. This can help in deciding how best to treat it.
- Please draw on the diagram below where you feel your pain. If you have pain in more than one area, **only shade in the one main area where your worst pain is.**

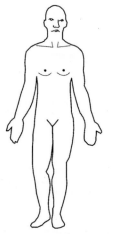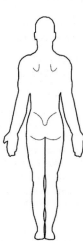

- On the scale below, please indicate how bad your pain (that you have shown on the above diagram) has been in the last week where: '0' means no pain and '10' means pain as severe as it could be.

NONE   0 1 2 3 4 5 6 7 8 9 10   **SEVERE PAIN**

- On the other side of the page are 7 questions about your pain (the one in the diagram).
- Think about how your pain that you showed in the diagram has felt **over the last week.** Put a tick against the descriptions that best match your pain. These descriptions may, or may not, match your pain, no matter how severe it feels.
- Only circle the responses that describe your pain. **Please turn over**.

S-LANSS

1. **In the area where you have pain, do you also have 'pins and needles', tingling, or prickling sensations?**

   a) NO – I don't get these sensations (0)

   b) YES – I get these sensations often (5)

2. **Does the painful area change colour (perhaps looks mottled or more red) when the pain is particularly bad?**

   a) NO – The pain does not affect the colour of my skin (0)

   b) YES – I have noticed that the pain does make my skin look different from normal (5)

3. **Does your pain make the affected skin abnormally sensitive to touch? Getting unpleasant sensations or pain when lightly stroking the skin might describe this.**

   a) NO – The pain does not make my skin in that area abnormally sensitive to touch (0)

   b) YES – My skin in that area is particularly sensitive to touch (3)

4. **Does your pain come on suddenly and in bursts for no apparent reason when you are completely still? Words like 'electric shocks', 'jumping', and 'bursting' might describe this.**

   a) NO – My pain doesn't really feel like this (0)

   b) YES – I get these sensations often (2)

5. **In the area where you have pain, does your skin feel unusually hot like a burning pain?**

   a) NO – I don't have burning pain (0)

   b) YES – I get burning pain often (1)

6. **Gently <u>rub</u> the painful area with your index finger and then rub a non-painful area (for example, an area of skin further away or on the opposite side from the painful area). How does this rubbing feel in the painful area?**

   a) The painful area feels no different from the non-painful area (0)

   b) I feel discomfort, like pins and needles, tingling, or burning in the painful area that is different from the non-painful area (5)

7. **Gently <u>press</u> on the painful area with your fingertip then gently press in the same way onto a non-painful area (the same non-painful area that you chose in the last question). How does this feel in the painful area?**

   a) The painful area does not feel different from the non-painful area (0)

   b) I feel numbness or tenderness in the painful area that is different from the non-painful area (3)

Scoring: a score of 12 or more suggests pain of predominantly neuropathic origin.

Neuropathic Pain Scale (NPS)

Galer, B.S. and Jensen, M.P. (1997). Development and preliminary validation of a pain measure specific to neuropathic pain: the Neuropathic Pain Scale. *Neurology*, **48**, 332–8.

The NPS is distributed through the MAPI website – www.mapi-research.fr/. The NPS is free to use in clinical practice but a fee is payable to use in funded research projects.

Neuropathic Pain Symptom Inventory (NPSI)

Bouhassira, D., Attal, N., Fermanian, J., Alchaar, H., Gautron, M., Masquelier, E., *et al.* (2004). Development and validation of the Neuropathic Pain Symptom Inventory. *Pain*, **108**, 248–57.

Douleur Neuropathique 4 (DN4)

Bouhassira, D., Attal, N., Alchaar, H., Boureau, F., Brochet, B., Bruxelle, J., *et al.* (2005). Comparison of pain syndromes associated with nervous or somatic lesions and development of a new neuropathic pain diagnostic questionnaire (DN4). *Pain*, **114**, 29–36.

Neuropathic Pain Questionnaire (NPQ)

Krause, S.J. and Backonja, M.M. (2003). Development of a neuropathic pain questionnaire. *Clin. J. Pain*, **19**, 306–14.

Index

W

V

Z